UNDERSTANDING SOCIOLOGY IN NURSING

HELEN ALLAN, MICHAEL TRAYNOR,
DANIEL KELLY AND PAM SMITH

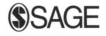

Los Angeles | London | New Delhi
Singapore | Washington DC | Melbourne

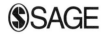

Los Angeles | London | New Delhi
Singapore | Washington DC | Melbourne

SAGE Publications Ltd
1 Oliver's Yard
55 City Road
London EC1Y 1SP

SAGE Publications Inc.
2455 Teller Road
Thousand Oaks, California 91320

SAGE Publications India Pvt Ltd
B 1/I 1 Mohan Cooperative Industrial Area
Mathura Road
New Delhi 110 044

SAGE Publications Asia-Pacific Pte Ltd
3 Church Street
#10-04 Samsung Hub
Singapore 049483

Editor: Becky Taylor
Editorial assistant: Charlène Burin
Production editor: Katie Forsythe
Copyeditor: Neil Dowden
Proofreader: Rosemary Campbell
Marketing manager: Camille Richmond
Cover design: Wendy Scott
Typeset by: C&M Digitals (P) Ltd, Chennai, India
Printed and bound in Great Britain by Bell and
Bain Ltd, Glasgow

Library of Congress Control Number: 2015951828

British Library Cataloguing in Publication data

A catalogue record for this book is available from
the British Library

ISBN 978-1-4739-1358-5
ISBN 978-1-4739-1359-2 (pbk)

At SAGE we take sustainability seriously. Most of our products are printed in the UK using FSC papers and boards.
When we print overseas we ensure sustainable papers are used as measured by the PREPS grading system.
We undertake an annual audit to monitor our sustainability.

UNDERSTANDI
SOCIOLOGY IN
N

SAGE was founded in 1965 by Sara Miller McCune to support the dissemination of usable knowledge by publishing innovative and high-quality research and teaching content. Today, we publish over 900 journals, including those of more than 400 learned societies, more than 800 new books per year, and a growing range of library products including archives, data, case studies, reports, and video. SAGE remains majority-owned by our founder, and after Sara's lifetime will become owned by a charitable trust that secures our continued independence.

Los Angeles | London | New Delhi | Singapore | Washington DC | Melbourne

Contents

About the authors

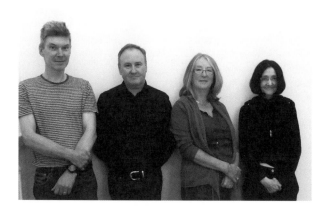

Helen Allan qualified as a nurse in 1978 at University College Hospital (UCH) and worked in various staff nurse posts (in acute care) until she decided she wanted to specialize in intensive care nursing. She completed her JBCNS 100 (ICU) at Guys Hospital, London and worked as a ward sister in intensive care at UCH from 1982–86.

She then went into education working as a clinical teacher, leaving to complete a BSc (Sociology) at the London School of Economics and Political Sciences, London, graduating in 1990. She completed her PGDE and registered as a nurse tutor in 1992, and starting work on her PhD while working as a nurse tutor in 1993. She graduated as a PhD in 1999.

Helen began her research career at the University of Surrey in 2001, had a brief interlude at York in 2013, before starting at Middlesex University in 2014. Her first Chair in Nursing was a joint appointment with the Royal Surrey County Hospital and subsequently she has held chairs at York and Middlesex. Helen has taught social sciences to nursing students pre and post registration for over 20 years and used her sociological insights into examining taken-for-grated assumptions about nursing practice over the same period.

Michael Traynor was born in London. Michael read English Literature at Cambridge, then completed general nursing and health visiting training. After working as a health visitor in London, he moved to Australia where he was a researcher for the South Australian Health Commission. Michael worked at the Royal College of Nursing in London from 1991 to 1996 and undertook a three-year study of nursing morale in the wake of the 1991 National Health Service reforms. Drawing on his background in literature, his PhD examined the language employed by nurses and their managers. It was published as a book by Routledge. He worked at the Centre for Policy in Nursing Research at the London School of Hygiene & Tropical Medicine. He is now Professor of Nursing Policy at Middlesex University in London. He researches professional identity and the application of discourse analysis and approaches from literary theory and psychoanalysis to nursing policy and healthcare issues. He is editor of the journal *Health: An Interdisciplinary Journal for the Social Study of Health, Illness and Medicine* and European editor of *Nursing Inquiry*. He recently wrote *Nursing in Context: Policy, Politics, Profession* published by Palgrave Macmillan.

Daniel Kelly undertook the integrated Social Sciences and Nursing degree at Edinburgh University. On qualifying in 1984 he worked in intensive care and trauma nursing before specializing in oncology. He undertook oncology training at The Royal Marsden hospital in London before returning to Edinburgh to take up two Charge Nurse posts in HIV and oncology. During this time he completed a masters degree in advanced cancer care. He returned to the Royal Marsden to teach cancer care for several years before moving to University College Hospitals as Senior Nurse for Research & Development. During this time he undertook a PhD in Sociology at Goldsmiths, University of London on the embodied impact of prostate cancer.

He has worked at a number of universities since then including City, Middlesex and Cardiff. His research interests have included cancer, end of life care, nursing innovation and more recently workplace culture and related factors such as leadership. He is Visiting Professorial Fellow in Nursing Studies at Edinburgh University and has been awarded a Churchill Fellowship. Underpinning this work has been an ongoing interest in sociology and the role of everyday behaviour in shaping healthcare practices.

Pam Smith is Professorial Fellow, Nursing Studies in the School of Health in Social Science, University of Edinburgh and a Visiting Professor in Nursing, King's College London. She is a graduate of the University of Manchester's Bachelor of Nursing programme where she qualified as a registered nurse, district nurse and health visitor (1970). Pam undertook postgraduate studies at London University where she obtained a certificate in adult education (Garnet College), an MSc in Medical Sociology (Bedford College) and her PhD on how student nurses learn to care (King's College). Pam worked as a nurse and teacher in Tanzania, Mozambique and Britain and as a nurse researcher in Britain and the USA. She spent 1989–90 with Professor Arlie Russell Hochschild at the University of California at Berkeley, developing the application of emotional labour to nursing. Former posts include Head of Nursing Studies, University of Edinburgh (2010–13), General Nursing Council Trust Chair in Nurse Education and Director of the Centre for Research in Nursing and Midwifery Education at the University of Surrey (2002–2008), Professor of Nursing, London South Bank University (1997–2001) and Director of Nursing Research and Development, Camden and Islington Health Authority (1988-92).

Pam's qualitative research includes collaborative studies of international aid and maternal and child health services in Nepal and Malawi; online education of maternal and child health professionals in Malawi; transitions from active to palliative care for children with cancer, parents and professionals; an exploration of the experiences of patients living with neuromuscular degenerative conditions and their families; patient safety and healthcare professional education; the UK experiences of overseas trained nurses; primary care and healthcare reform.

Pam is the author of *The Emotional Labour of Nursing: How Nurses Care* (1992: Palgrave Macmillan) and *The Emotional Labour of Nursing Revisited: Can Nurses Still Care?* (2012: Palgrave Macmillan).

Foreword

This book is an excellent introduction to how clinical work can be understood as affected by particular social and cultural forces. It helps foreground not just how nurses train and work in complex environments – the normal chaos of healthcare services under strain – but how important it is to understand that these environments are also deeply structured.

Nurses are never ever free to do whatever they choose. So many clinical textbooks represent nurses as autonomous decision-makers with the discretion to conduct care in line with standards and protocols decided far from the plane of action, providing they have the right education, knowledge, skills and experience. What these ways of representing nursing leave out is how nursing is conducted in environments that are complex, prefigured by social and cultural, not just clinical or bioethical, values. For example, nursing is entangled in cultural preoccupations that privilege some kinds of knowledge and work, such as highly techno-medical work, and that deface other kinds of knowledge and work, for example 'body' or 'care' work. In addition nurses are continuously being positioned by multiple and often competing agendas. For example those carried by an audit culture which intensifies the need to be seen to meet particular targets rather than the needs and cares of an individual patient. As the Francis Report amongst others has put it, it is as if nurses are being asked to care more for the system, including extremely limited ideas about efficiency, than for their patients.

Sociology is concerned with helping illuminate this complexity and its unintended consequences. It also helps us to see all the invisible and often neglected patching and knitting work that nurses do to make these complex environments run at all. And that's what this book helps do. It helps us to see how to draw in different theoretical positions not just to make sense of the complexity but to illuminate the aspects of being a nurse and doing nursing, and of becoming ill and being a patient, that remain invisible if we only examine them from a biomedical or even a psychological perspective.

It is in this respect that I appreciate the way that the book grounds discussion and explication of key sociological ideas in the everyday worlds of nursing students' experience, helping to illuminate how this is rooted in the social, cultural and political conditions of contemporary healthcare. Here the book draws on examples from each authors' extensive repertoires of empirical research as well as a vast array of literature across key domains: being a patient, becoming a nurse and doing nursing, the social construction of health and illness, the gendering of nursing and the division of healthcare labour, the meanings of care, patient safety and organisational complexity, the body and emotional labour, and the problems with discourses of leadership and technologies of management.

The book will not only help nurses to think critically about how and why they work in the ways that they do but will empower them to do things differently. For a long time sociology has been a core subject in medical education. I have long argued it should be a core subject for nurse education. This erudite but eminently accessible book should be compulsory reading on every undergraduate nursing programme.

Joanna Latimer, Professor of Sociology,
Science & Technology, University of York.

Introduction

Helen Allan, Daniel Kelly, Pam Smith and Michael Traynor

Why me?

Our daily experiences as individuals are, to an extent that would surprise the unsuspecting, determined by an array of social forces – all the more so for those like you who are working in the complex environment of healthcare work. Some of these forces are stable and long established, such as the effects of gender, while others are highly unpredictable and changing even as you read this book, like the rise of social media (which we discuss in Chapter 3). Perhaps reassuringly, many of these have been noted and investigated from different perspectives. In this book we will be looking at the work of sociologists. Their accounts offer us explanations for apparently contradictory events and experiences such as the tension of trying to deliver individualised care while being responsible for the flow of patients through a ward or unit and the meeting of organisational requirements. It is the goal of this book to encourage you to think about these kinds of experiences from a sociological perspective.

Why sociology?

Sociology is the study of human social life, groups and societies. Sociologists study everything from everyday interactions, which are usually taken for granted, to global issues, such as how countries and cultures come into conflict.

Sociology emerged in the nineteenth century as philosophers and scientists developed explanations or theories for the huge social changes that swept Western Europe. A key figure in early sociological thought, Auguste Comte (1798–1857), endeavoured to 'discover' social facts in the same way as biologists and psychologists such as Darwin and Freud were later to do within their disciplines. For Comte, sociology was the 'queen of the sciences'. He thought sociology should answer questions about why people in groups, that is of more than two or three, behave in the way they do. Was their behaviour predetermined in any way? What were the social rules of groups and how were these passed down over generations?

We see nursing and healthcare as essentially social activities that can be analysed from the perspective of how the individuals involved are influenced by the social world around them. Sociology offers you a way of understanding what is happening, for example, when you join a group such as your cohort of fellow students. It can also help you to understand the organisation of work you encounter in clinical placements and develop understanding of patients' experiences of illness. By focusing on everyday events, sociology makes the ordinary extraordinary and can reveal to us hidden reasons why people do what they do. This includes the way that you learn to 'become a nurse' and a member of different subgroups along the way.

Unlike other books presenting a broad range of sociological ideas to nurses, we take as our starting point the issues that nurses experience from day to day and build links from these issues to the social theory that can help in understanding them. In the process we will introduce you to key concepts, debates and thinkers in sociology. These can shed light on the experiences you might go through, in different environments, with different people while learning to do many different things. Many health professions share the requirement for those entering the profession to simultaneously learn and work. This sometimes involves a delicate balance. Having a structure and some theories[1] to bring to bear on the complexity of our study and working lives can free us from simply reacting to the problems and uncertainties we face and can provide us with a source of critical resilience. Social theories help explain sets of social conditions or types of occurrences and can help suggest solutions to particular types of social problems. Many nurses express a sense of relief to find that they are not alone in experiencing feelings of uncertainty or anxiety about how to act in certain situations. In this book we draw on situations that may be common to many nursing students and use these to raise points for you to think about or debate in groups. As you do so, we encourage you to think of the social processes that shape people's attitudes, beliefs and behaviour, including your own. For example, Scenario 1 shows you how the social process of being a student can be reflected upon and used productively.

---

[1]A theory can be defined in a number of ways: as an explanatory framework, a set of abstract or generalised statements about a topic derived (often but not always) from observations or the building up of a body of knowledge.

Scenario 1

It was great being there with newly qualified nurses ... to go 'I just don't get it', 'which anti-hypertensive can you give before theatre', 'which ones [you] can't' and everyone else going 'ah, I've heard a little trick for that' or 'yeah, the way you want to think about that' ...

This quote comes from a research study Helen has undertaken into how senior students learn to work as newly qualified nurses. The speaker is a newly qualified nurse. Her learning was clearly improved by sharing her anxieties about her new role with her peers.

For advice on how to use scenarios, see below.

Summary of chapters

Chapters 1 and 2 deal with patients: how people become patients and who patients are. We argue in Chapter 1 that part of the process of becoming a patient involves 'learning' about the role. Although taking on 'the sick role' might temporarily excuse you from certain expectations such as turning up for work, there are, increasingly, other requirements such as a willingness to do what is needed to get better. This can extend to taking responsibility for your own health and, in the case of chronic disease, such as diabetes, for monitoring your own condition. Some patient groups, for example those diagnosed with HIV/AIDS or with mental health problems, have mounted challenges to the idea that patients should remain docile recipients of medical care. At a more detailed level, patients learn how to talk to health professionals in particular ways to maximise the chances of getting the care they want and to exercise some control. In Chapter 2 we discuss the social forces that are at work influencing the patterns of health and illness among different groups and in different locations. Rather than seeing these patterns of inequality as being completely determined, we offer the opportunity to understand why they occur and what can be done to challenge them. We also discuss examples of what some nurses, in partnership with patients, have been able to do about them. In these two chapters we use the concept of 'macro' and 'micro' to understand the interplay of societal forces with individual and group experience. By 'macro' sociology we mean the study of social forces or structures such as capitalism and social processes such as class, gender and ethnicity. 'Micro' sociology is the study of face-to-face social interactions between people or groups (Dillon, 2010).

In Chapter 3 of this book we look at what happens to people when they become nurses. At one level those training to be nurses are taught a range of skills and there are attempts to instil so-called professional values such as respect for patients, but there is much more going on. Those entering any profession learn informally how to respond and behave as members of that profession. However, nursing and healthcare professionals are unlike other professions because they deal, on a daily basis, with aspects of living and dying that the majority of people would never encounter during their working lives. So, just to take one example, those becoming nurses learn to routinise events, such as bathing a patient who is essentially a stranger, which those outside the profession would find unacceptable. Because this learning and changing, though informal, is more or less shared, we can talk about 'professional socialisation'. In this chapter we will also discuss the usefulness of social media for those becoming nurses.

In Chapter 4 we analyse nursing work in terms of patriarchy, demographic characteristics of nurses and the healthcare workforce more widely in terms of hierarchy, power and the division of labour. In the final section of the chapter we consider some of the strategies some nurses use to resist, assert and overcome domination, oppression and scapegoating. These strategies play an important role not only when things go wrong (see Chapter 7) but also to prevent things going wrong in the first place. Strategies include joining unions, professional organisations, forming pressure groups, and developing unique nursing knowledge and innovative practice such as the 'new nursing' initiatives described in Chapter 6.

In Chapter 5 we focus on emotions and care, suggesting theoretical frameworks that can help you understand the part they play in nursing work. Some suggest that nurses are expected to manage their emotions irrespective of the personal costs and this can result in stress and burnout. As you progress through your programme, you may be exposed to many different situations giving rise to responses ranging from optimism and reward to withdrawal and exhaustion. To examine this further, we draw on work by sociologist Arlie Hochschild (1983) who developed the concept of 'emotional labour' to describe the invisible, unrewarded work involved in the service sector, that is in 'people work'. The concept of emotional labour draws on the fundamental sociological concepts of 'structure' and 'agency'. 'Structure' is the recurrent patterned arrangements that influence or limit the choices and opportunities available to people. Agency is the capacity of individuals to act independently and make their own choices (Giddens, 1984).

Chapter 6 focuses on care of the body in nursing. Much of the work undertaken by nurses involves some level of contact with illness. This is most immediately obvious in the effect on the body of the sick individual. As a student nurse you will be expected to deal with aspects of the human body and its functions normally kept private or viewed with some distaste. This could include dealing with a body after death. Nurses deal with the aged, traumatised or 'out of control' body, which can present a troubling spectacle and a challenge for nurses, especially for those who are new to this work. Whilst this kind of care is very important to patients and families, it may be seen as lower status and relegated to the least qualified worker. Sociologists have also considered the importance of the body through a range of issues such as sexuality and the stigma associated with certain conditions such as infectious diseases and eating disorders.

Given the reality of nursing – its highly pressured place in a complex health service under continual political and media pressure – it is not surprising that sometimes things go wrong. The early years of the 2010s have seen particular high-profile 'exposures' of healthcare-system failures in the UK National Health Service. Everyone, it seems, has an explanation about what is wrong but we encourage you to consider where some of these reasons are uninformed and somewhat simplistic. Chapter 7 discusses not only the complex factors that can contribute to failures of care, but also asks why nurses are so often scapegoated by politicians, journalists and others. A key focus of this chapter will be the Francis Inquiry Report from 2013 (Francis, 2013).

As a student nurse you will have experienced different leadership styles and you will have your own views about what makes good leadership. In Chapter 8 we encourage you to reflect on the importance of effective leadership and management in shaping the culture of care. When things have gone wrong in nursing and healthcare it is often put down to poor leadership. Chapter 8 discusses the multi-million pound phenomenon of the leadership industry. It examines how healthcare managers and clinical professionals may have conflicting interests within National Health Service (NHS) organisations. This chapter also sets out some theories of power and so-called styles of leadership. It concludes by discussing the opportunities that nurses have to exercise leadership and challenge the status quo.

Chapter 9 concludes the book and, by taking lessons from each chapter, offers a sociological understanding for your own working situation, for changing it, or for surviving it in an intelligent and critical way. This ability will we hope provide resilience – critical resilience – throughout your career.

How to use this book

It is customary for authors of textbooks to give suggestions to students about how to use their books. Please feel free to read the chapters in any order. In most chapters we have include printed links to Internet web pages in order to illustrate points we are making or provide interesting further reading. Please consider taking the trouble to type these into a computer browser to visit these sites. We have also included some boxes in each chapter which contain points at which to reflect on your own experiences (reflections) or practice scenarios to provoke further thought and begin to do this from a sociological viewpoint.

Every chapter opens with a current issue which we use as a springboard to introduce key sociological thinkers and their associated theories.

This book is a collaboration of four people. We have worked hard to make sure we do not contradict each other but you will detect different voices behind different chapters. We hope that will make the book more interesting. We have generally used 'we' to make our arguments, though when one of us is writing about their own experiences or research projects we have used 'I'.

References

Dillon, M. (2010) *Introduction to Sociological Theory: Theorists, Concepts and Their Applicability to the Twenty-First Century*. Chichester: Wiley-Blackwell.

Francis, R. (2013) *Report of the Mid Staffordshire NHS Foundation Trust Public Inquiry: Executive Summary*. London: House of Commons, HC 947.

Giddens A. (1984) *The Constitution of Society*. Berkeley, CA: University of California Press.

Hochschild A.R. (1983) *The Managed Heart: Commercialisation of Human Feeling*. Berkeley, CA: University of California Press.

1

Becoming a patient

Helen Allan

Issue

The sociological issue that is the focus of this chapter is what happens when you – or your parent, child or friend – become a patient.

Read the following scenario and reflect on your responses.

Scenario 1.1

Imagine you are admitted to hospital to a day surgery ward for an investigation. It is early in the morning; you have not had breakfast, a cup of tea or even a drink of water. You are worried, even scared, of what is going to happen as you have heard the procedure is uncomfortable.

You have been asked to leave any valuables at home which includes your wedding ring, earrings and other jewellery. You are asked to change into a hospital gown and given a pair of rather horrid paper knickers. And then you wait ... for ages it seems although it might only be 15 minutes before someone comes over to say they will be back to ask you some questions. You're not sure who they are as they're wearing an ill-fitting blue top and trousers which you suppose is what they wear in theatres but it doesn't help you understand who they are.

How could you be made to feel more at ease? Do you have to be stripped of all your personal possessions?

What could the staff do to reduce your anxiety and make you feel less scared?

While it may be necessary to prepare patients for surgery in the way described above, nevertheless becoming a patient may not just involve a loss of dignity but the gradual erosion of your identity as you conform to the expectations of those who are caring for you. Does being a patient mean that you suddenly become subject to the hospital's rules and regulations? Do you *have* to have your temperature taken every four hours? Are you treated as if you make the decisions? What happens if you disagree with your doctor, nurse or physiotherapist? Can you complain and what happens to complaints anyway? Sometimes as nurses we expect patients to behave in ways which aren't always necessary and may involve a loss of rights to autonomy or dignity.

It is also worth noting that while the example above is a hospital-based one, the issues we discuss in this chapter, and indeed throughout the book, apply to all patients in a range of contexts such as mental health settings and community settings as well as learning disability.

How people learn to become patients (Revans, 1964) has interested sociologists for a long time and is a good illustration of macro and micro sociology. Some of the theories, such as the sick role, you might have come across; others won't be so well known. The chapter finishes with a discussion of patient-centred care which is, in our view, a logical development from macro to micro sociological approaches to understanding how people become patients.

Chapter outline

The chapter is divided into three broad sections:

- Macro sociology
  - The sick role and the social system
- Micro sociology
  - When the patient encounters the doctor
  - The subjective experience of being a patient
  - Narratives/patient stories
- Patient-centred care
  - What do patients want?
  - Patient surveys

Macro sociology

Structural functionalism: the sick role as a social process and healthcare as a social system

Earlier in the last century, sociologists, in particular American sociologist Talcott Parsons (1902–79), called this learning process *taking on 'the sick role'*; that is, a person who is unwell or ill is allowed to adopt a role and concomitant behaviours that might temporarily excuse them from certain expectations such as turning up for work. Note I say *allowed* – this is important because Parsons was interested in how individuals functioned in society and contributed to the functioning of that society; in the main their roles as employees and in the family. He was therefore interested in what mechanisms existed to allow them time off from work. So adults are expected to work until retirement unless there are very good reasons why not. Illness was one of those mechanisms that allowed the individual to take time off work; other mechanisms are paid holidays or retirement. But illness was also not normal behaviour, rather a sort of *deviance*, as, by being ill, individuals did not conform to society's expectations, albeit temporarily. Of course this model depends on the patient presenting with recognisable symptoms and signs that the doctor then diagnoses. At this point the doctor can refer the patient for tests or to a specialist. However, sometimes the doctor doesn't recognise the illness, mistrusts the patient's story, and irrespective of whether the patient continues to experience symptoms, there is then a possibility that the patient will not be signed off and not be validated as being sick. In other words, diagnosing illness is not straightforward.

Read Reflection 1.1 in the box below and reflect on your thoughts about the doctor's role in legitimating the sick role.

Reflection 1.1

Think of how people suffering from myalgic encephalomyelitis (ME) struggled to have their symptoms recognised as a legitimate illness – it is often referred to as chronic fatigue syndrome, which patients believe underplays how serious an illness it is and the effects on lives it can have.

Have a look at the website of the ME Association: www.meassociation.org. uk/2007/01/overview/.

What do you think the note on the website signifies? 'PLEASE NOTE – before considering prognosis, it is important to obtain a positive diagnosis, which should be determined only by a suitably qualified medical professional.'

I think this statement is a good example of the power of the doctor to diagnose. It upholds the idea of the sick role and the expectation that an individual should not self-diagnose as diagnosis remains in the hands of doctors.

The idea of society functioning as a system dependent on its parts was very much a feature of the USA and the UK in the 1950s. Illness was one way for an adult to get sanctioned time off work as long as it was certified by a doctor. Therefore the doctor becomes an agent of social control; in fact, 'The sick role is, for Parsons, one of the most important mechanisms of social control in capitalist societies' (Varul, 2010: 76).

The social system

In *The Social System* (1951), Parsons said that the doctor–patient relationship was functional for society because it meant that people could be off sick, diagnosed by a doctor and then cured (or if they had a chronic disease, be managed by a doctor over a longer period). This concern with function or roles within society is described in sociology as structural functionalism.

Parsons believed that individuals' behaviours need to be understood as social behaviours rather than as determined by individuals' internal processes or cognitions (which is what psychologists study). He advocated the study of the social systems in which people lived; in other words, the social structures and cultural values that both constrained and facilitated action and behaviours.

Concern among sociologists about the nature of social structures and individual agency, the collective perspective or the individual, was first written about by nineteenth-century sociologists. Karl Marx (1818–1883), Emile Durkheim (1858–1917) and Max Weber (1864–1920) were all writing about this topic at roughly the same time, the mid to late nineteenth century and the early twentieth century. They all took different views of how strong either structure or the individual (agency) was in reproducing social norms, values and behaviours; in producing society.

Durkheim was interested in the functioning of specific social structures, such as crime and religion, while Weber studied the social actions of individuals that were influenced by their values and the economic system in which they lived (capitalism essentially). Parsons, born after Marx, Durkheim and Weber, but drawing on their work and the work of Freud, a psychologist, was more interested in social structures: in the social system (society), social institutions such as universities and social structures such as healthcare, and their functional roles in maintaining the equilibrium of society, the social order or the status quo.

The doctor–patient relationship

The doctor–patient relationship is part of a social sub-system that kicks into action when there is a 'disturbance of normal functioning of the total human individual' (Parsons, 1951: 431–432), as Parsons called illness or disease. So when an individual is functioning normally, their body and mind function normally also and they do not have any need of the doctor. When their body or mind (their total human individual) begins to malfunction, then individuals become patients and are required to seek out the doctor. This is because illness threatens society by depriving it of the particular function of the individual. For example, the mother or father who is sick cannot care for her or his children's needs; the nurse cannot care for their patients. Illness therefore is a social phenomenon not an individual one. That imposes duties on the patient to report illness and to follow any treatment while at the same time imposing on the doctor the duty to treat the patient and on society to look after anyone diagnosed as ill. This is the reason you have to have a certificate from your doctor to show your employer and also why you are entitled to sick pay while off sick. Parsons calls this a social contract between the individual in society who becomes the patient seeking help from the doctor, who has a duty to care for him or her.

Of course there are critiques of Parsons' theory, not least because he seems to talk about acute illness not chronic illness although his model is applied to chronic illness now (see Varul, 2010). He also seems to reinforce gender norms (the doctor is invariably male). And his model assumes that an individual has a doctor to go to. How does Parsons' sick role apply to homeless people or migrant workers who are not registered with general practitioners in the UK? Lastly, and by no means least, Parsons' theory is based on a Western, twentieth-century model of health and medicine.

Critiques of Parsons' sick role

The most obvious criticism is that Parsons was writing about a Westernised health-care system. In other countries and social systems, expectations about the 'sick role' are not so prevalent or may not exist at all and there may be other expectations and sanctions in place. This becomes evident when patients access the British health system and the welfare state more generally for the first time. They may be used to different value systems in both the doctor's consultation and in relation to the role of the state in providing benefits for sick leave. Consequently these patients may have difficulties navigating or even understanding the requirements expected of them or the benefits available.

You might have noticed that the doctor in Parsons' model is the active partner in the doctor–patient relationship and he[1] has all the power; to diagnose and legitimate illness for example, to 'sign' someone off from work. The patient actively adopts the sick role, but once they have entered into their relationship with their doctor, they are passive in the relationship. In other words, they surrender the responsibilities otherwise generally expected of them by society. According to Parsons, patients are passive recipients of doctors' (and nurses') care and have few other responsibilities apart from taking their medicine[2] and obeying the doctor.

Reflection 1.2

Think about the idea that patients are passive for a moment:
Why are they? Are they all passive? Does this make them powerless and the doctor powerful? What conditions make it easier for patients to be assertive?
What does the sick role model imply for the nurse–patient relationship? Who has power in the nurse–patient relationship?
Is this power relationship shifting?
How do you feel about this?
Patients as well as having the right to become active in their treatment also have the right to choose a more passive position within their relationships with clinicians, doctors, nurses or therapists. This is not passivity in the form of disempowerment or as Parsons was describing, but may exist as a conscious informed choice. See Going Further section below for some additional reading on Arnstein's Ladder of Participation.

---

[1]Note that Parsons' model of the sick role was gendered, i.e. he spoke invariably about male doctors. This reflected relationships between men and women and gender roles in 1950s America (Varul, 2010).

[2]Although it must be said that the medicine cupboard was kept locked by the nurse who worked with the doctor and in some sense was invested with authority and power from their association with the doctor.

You can see how Parsons' sick-role model might not work today when patients are encouraged to be far more responsible for their own health. The model is also based on a sense of shared values, namely an acceptance that the doctor has power. But the sick-role model might exclude individuals or groups who challenge these 'shared' values, for example gays, lesbians, people of black and ethnic minority backgrounds. Imagine yourself as an unemployed, black man who heard voices. What would the doctor say to you? Would the doctor recognise your cultural beliefs if they were contrary to the majority white population?

Reflection 1.3

Have a look at this website: www.hearing-voices.org/targetgroup/bme-communities.

Try reading Hari Sewell's *Working with Ethnicity, Race and Culture in Mental Health: A Handbook for Practitioners*. It gives an overview of how much power doctors have historically had over patients and particularly over patients from black and minority ethnic (BME) backgrounds.

We will discuss these issues of inequalities in the next chapter.

Another important critique of the structural functionalist view of society is that it tends to locate power as a variable sum; that is, power is held by individuals in relation to the role they hold within society for the benefit of society. So doctors hold power once patients consult them, for everyone's benefit. This is different to Marx and Weber who thought of power as a constant sum. In other words, power is held by one group at the expense of another. There's only so much power to go around (Wilkinson, 1999). Additionally, power may be used by some to further their own interests. Now this last view is clearly not part of Parsons' model of the professional role of doctors; Parsons assumes doctors act for the benefit of society as a whole (as above). But equally, in the doctor–patient relationship, power is located with the doctor as s/he has the power to validate the patients' symptoms and define them as signs of disease.

Reflection 1.4

How far do you think the nurse–patient relationship mirrors the doctor–patient relationship as Parsons describes it?

Power and nursing

Very importantly, Parsons' model didn't recognise the nursing role; that the nurse had the medicine cabinet key (see above) didn't mean she had power necessarily.

However, that doesn't mean to say that nurses were not an important part of the patient experience of healthcare at the time Parsons was writing, the 1950s–1960s. Studies have shown that nurses were powerful at this time (see Chapter 3). Unfortunately, studies have also shown that nurses didn't challenge the sick role and used it in some ways to collude with the disempowerment of mental health patients (Roger et al., 1993). So nurses worked to advance their own position with medicine and, as Roger et al. show, against patients' interests rather than work with patients.

Others have criticised the strategy nurses use to build powerful positions within healthcare as managers and as handmaidens of the medical profession (Garmarnikov, 1978). As far as we're concerned in this chapter, this is important to understanding becoming a patient because patients need to know who runs the show, who will organise their care, who makes the decisions and understands their situation and who is aware of them as a person (Allan, 2002; Allan and Barber 2005).

Lastly, and we will discuss this in more detail in Chapter 2 when we consider health inequalities, Parsons did not discuss in his writings that society instead of being beneficent could actually be making us ill.

We will now move on to micro sociological approaches which have also been present in sociological theory since the late nineteenth century. Before we do we will consider two events that have profoundly influenced being a patient since Parsons first wrote 'Illness and the role of physicians: a sociological perspective' in 1975.

1. On the one hand, from the 1980s onwards, some patient groups, for example those diagnosed with HIV/AIDS or with mental health problems, have mounted challenges to the idea of the sick role and argued that patients should not remain docile recipients of medical care. Other groups of patients who challenged the sick role were women's health groups and the disabled, who wished in particular not to be seen as *sick* but as living with a disability. Patients were empowered to talk to health professionals in particular ways to maximise the chances of getting the care they wanted and to exercise some control.

2. On the other hand, there are increasingly expectations and, sometimes, even requirements brought to bear on the patient on being diagnosed, such as a willingness to do what is needed to get better. This can extend to taking responsibility for your own health and, in the case of chronic disease such as diabetes, for monitoring your own condition.

Consequently, the relationships that shape the patient experience of being a patient, the doctor–patient relationship, the doctor–nurse relationship and the nurse–patient relationship, have undergone dramatic change over the last 30 years. Arthur Frank, an American sociologist working in this area, described the change in emphasis from macro sociology to micro sociology as *listening to patients* and said this started in the 1980s:

> Sociologists of my generation [i.e. born in the 1930s/1940s] talked mostly to physicians, occasionally to nurses, rarely to patients. The idea of the ill patient as someone living with serious illness but having a life beyond medical treatment was an innovation of the 1980s. (Frank, 2014)

I expect the idea of talking to patients is second nature to you as students in healthcare now; but it wasn't if you trained before the 1980s and the sick role has remained influential until recently. The shift Frank talks about from medical sociology (the study of medicine largely) to a sociology of health and illness was both prompted by and based on an acknowledgement of patient power, patient perspectives that have dramatically altered the role and responsibilities of both the doctor/nurse and the patient. It also led to the resurgence of micro-sociology approaches in influencing health delivery.

Micro sociology

Micro-sociological theories can help us understand *becoming a patient* through their focus on when the patient encounters the doctor and the subjective experience of being a patient. Sociologists have always been interested in the experience of the individual; Weber, for example, articulated the concept of *verstehen* – understanding meaningful action. Only human beings are capable of meaningful action – action that is *intended* because of our relationships with and to other human beings (and of course other objects). He said (paraphrased of course) 'you can count the number of trees a man cuts down, but you need to understand why he cuts them down'. In nursing, we could say 'we can count the number of times an obese child eats the wrong sugary treat, but we need to understand why she does so to effect change in her diet'.

From Weber's work, two broad areas of theory have developed since the late nineteenth century, namely symbolic interactionism and phenomenology. We will consider ethnomethodology in Chapter 3, which is another important micro-sociological theory.

When the patient encounters the doctor

When the patient first meets the doctor, they bring with them ideas about what a patient does in a consultation, what a doctor does; what sorts of feelings are appropriate and what are not; even what might be appropriate clothing, level of cleanliness; what might be appropriate to say in front of a younger doctor or a female doctor? These ideas come from previous consultations, other people's experiences and exposure to the media and literature. They are built on interactions of one sort or another. *Symbolic interactionism* helps us understand these social interactions in a way that macro sociology doesn't.

So what does symbolic interactionism mean? Interactionism is concerned with how individuals and groups interact; so for our purposes, how do 'doctor Jones' and 'patient Hannah' interact? What can we observe about how they stand, sit, the language each use, the conversational turn taking and who appears to dominate the interaction?

Symbolic interactionism is a way of understanding social interactions through the meaning individuals in those interactions give to their actions before, during and after. We use the words *before*, *during* and *after* on purpose because we wish to convey the need to understand the interaction *in* the moment, as it happens, and also understand it once it's over or even before it happens. This builds on Weber's idea of *verstehen*, knowing why the patient is not taking his medication as much as the number of times he doesn't take it. These ideas might be familiar to you or you might have been introduced to them as part of reflection in your under graduate programme, even to the idea of what Schon (1983) calls reflection in action and reflection on action. However, reflection is sometimes an isolated, individually constructed experience.

Meaning for symbolic interactionists is never individually constructed; meaning is always co-constructed. 'The meaning of a thing for a person grows out of the ways in which other persons act toward the person with regard to the thing' (Blumer, 1962: 4–5)

The self

George Mead (1863–1931), an American sociologist, is thought of as the 'father of symbolic interactionism'; he was interested in the self – namely, how we reflected on ourselves and our actions as objects not just as subjects. So if we feel pain, it is subjective pain. But it is also objective; we say how much it hurts, we describe it if asked and we can tell others about it. In this way we are reflexive – or we are able to reflect. Mead argued that we learnt as children to be reflexive and to reflect on ourselves. Charles Cooley (1864–1929), who was Mead's student, argued that the self can only develop through interactions with others; it is through others that we develop our sense of self – the *looking-glass self* (Dillon, 2010).

But why symbolic? We each have individual meaning which we attribute to actions but as we develop a looking-glass self, a self constructed through interactions and validation from others, then we also construct shared meanings which in time take on symbolic meaning; that is, we don't need to constantly repeat what we mean when we eat a meal together. In certain circumstances it's shorthand for intimacy and love. It symbolises these concepts. Herbert Blumer (1900–1987), another American sociologist, put it much more eloquently, talking of:

> the peculiar and distinctive character of interaction as it takes place between human beings. The peculiarity consists in the fact that human beings interpret or define each other's actions instead of merely reacting to each other's actions. Their 'response' is not made directly to the actions of one another but instead is based on the meaning which they attach to such actions. Thus human interaction is mediated by the use of symbols, by interpretation or by ascertaining the meaning of one another's actions. (1962: 180)

Awareness of dying: Glaser and Strauss

An example in health research of symbolic interactionism is Glaser and Strauss' work on death and dying in hospitals, first published as *Awareness of Dying*. Glaser and Strauss were interested in the social interactions between nurses, doctors and patients in modern hospitals, and the use of technology and how patients were cared for, particularly when they were dying. Their book *Awareness of Dying* was a ground-breaking study for two reasons: first, instead of testing an existing social theory, they used empirical data to construct a new theory of dying in hospitals, which was later published as the grounded theory method (1965) (Chamberlain-Salaun et al., 2013). Grounded theory is a very popular research methodology in nursing and you might be familiar with Glaser and Strauss' work from research methods. Second, and importantly, they showed how dying was constructed through everyday interactions between doctors, medical teams, nurses and patients within the hospital, and what meanings were attributed to both artefacts, in this case hospital equipment or technologies, and symbols encompassed within these interactions. Although written about 20 years later, Strauss' paper 'Sentimental work in the technologized hospital', in which he and his colleagues set out how technology in large hospitals shapes the doctor–patient relationship and therefore being a patient, remains influential in nursing and palliative care.

Labelling theory and deviancy

An influential development within symbolic interactionism for mental health nursing was Irving Goffman's work on stigma. Goffman (1922–1982) studied mental illness and the institutions *mental asylums* in which patients with mental illness were incarcerated in the mid-twentieth century. Before we discuss stigma we need to revisit the shared nature of symbolic interactions and Becker's ideas around *deviance*.

Goffman's work on stigma built on the suggestion of Howard Becker (born 1928) that certain situations were considered in different societies to be shameful, polluting and deviant; they evoked feelings of disgust and/or shame because they broke expectations of social norms. People, including the affected person, assigned a negative meaning to the affected self.

Reflection 1.5

AIDS is a good example of a disease that evokes stigma, disgust and avoidance – look at the AVERT website: www.avert.org/hiv-aids-stigma-and-discrimination.htm.

You could also watch a powerful advert that was responsible for the increase in prejudice and fear of AIDS: www.youtube.com/watch?v=TMnb 536WuC0.

Can you think of other conditions either in nursing or in the wider society that evoke disgust?

Widowhood and sexual violence are a couple: www.widowsforpeace.org/war-widowhood-sexual-violence-stigma-displacement-and-poverty/.

Perhaps infertility: www.who.int/bulletin/volumes/88/12/10-011210/en/.

Even adoption: www.jstor.org/discover/10.2307/585831?uid=3739256&uid=2129&uid=2&uid=70&uid=4&sid=21105372031453.

How might you challenge these prejudices? This video clip gives one individual's response to social stigma: www.bbc.co.uk/news/magazine-33381431.

Becker argued that society *labelled* these states or conditions; he called this labelling theory.

A nursing example might be malignant fungating wounds (Lo et al., 2008) which evoke disgust and shame in both the patient and others around; this disgust may be evoked by smell, visible leakage or a misshapen body perhaps caused by wound dressings.

Becker argues this is because the meaning attributed to the wound by the patient and others with whom the patient interacts constructs a shared meaning.

Scenario 1.2   Living with a urinary catheter

Alison Chapple uses Goffmann's symbolic interactionism to understand living with a urinary catheter. She uses Goffman to suggest that incontinence is deviant as it breaks expectations around smell and bodily function, and is disrespectful to others. But it is created by the self (the patient) and others they interact with; they all construct meaning to label the deviancy.

www.healthtalk.org/files/nursing_times_living-with-an-indwelling-urinary-catheter.pdf.

So what is stigma? Labelling theory was applied to mental health by Scheff (1974: 25) to explain psychiatric symptoms as 'labelled violations of social norms'. For many of us, social norms are implicit, shared, residual rules that we take care not to break, such as not listening to other people's conversations or table manners. Scheff (born 1929) pointed out that for psychiatric patients, their behaviours were broken residual rules which had been labelled by society as deviant and 'mad'. Of course these rules change across societies and over time; what might be a rule yesterday isn't a rule today. Using a napkin properly when eating springs to mind or proper grammar in emails and texts. The rule breaker is then labelled as deviant, as psychiatric, and begins a deviant career.

Mental illness as a career

Goffman applied the idea of career in the sense of a moral career (not an occupational one) to the mentally ill patient. He identified stages through which the patient passed in this career, which begins with others deciding that the patient needs psychiatric care, then the patient is admitted to hospital and undergoes a loss of identity – who they are becomes stripped away as they lose their rights of independence. Goffman argued that the patient enters a total institution where the usual rights and privileges are removed and the self is further lost from sight. Goffman called this the mortification of the self. For further reading on Goffman's ideas about the total institution and the career of a mental health patient, read Benny Goodman's 2013 editorial on the application of Goffman's total institution to the state of nursing today.

Stigma

Having considered the concepts underpinning stigma, we can now discuss it. Building on symbolic interactionist ideas around a label assigning meaning (negative or discrediting), Goffman suggested that mental health patients acquired a stigmatising label from interactions with others, which has consequences (from the negative meaning) for the labelled individual. This was known as stigma. So an example might be a woman who has a sexually acquired disease from being a sex worker. For Goffman this occupation and the resulting disease means that this woman (or patient if we meet her in a clinic) is stigmatised both by herself and by others; that is, she does not meet society's expectations of women's roles or stereotypes. The stigma means that she has to work hard to convince us that she's a good woman despite the stigma. None of this is articulated; it is a shared meaning, a symbol that as members of society we all understand. Goffman calls this impression management. I've given an example above that is not so common in everyday life but all of us do impression management according to Goffman; I do it to maintain the impression that I am a functioning academic, a working mother and a good cook! But the stigma or the label attached to being a poor cook isn't so serious as that attached to being a sex worker or a woman with a sexually transmitted disease. The bigger the difference between the stereotype of the expected and the actual behaviour, the more the individual has to do impression management. Unfortunately, the more stigma is attached to the situation or condition, the more shame the individual also experiences.

I've said that Goffman wrote about stigma in connection with mental health. However, in other areas of illness, stigma is frequently experienced along with shame. For example, we have suggested malignant fungating wounds and sexual health. Some cancers are also stigmatising, along with many forms of disability.

Subjective experience of being a patient

Our second micro approach to sociological theory is *phenomenology* which is concerned with intersubjectivity, meaning and the life world.

Edmund Husserl (1859–1938) was a mathematician who originally focused on explaining an absolute foundation of philosophy in consciousness, without any presuppositions except what can be found through the reflective analysis of consciousness and what is immediately present to it. Originally, all judgements of the real were to be 'bracketed' or suspended, and then analysed to bring to light the role of consciousness in constituting or constructing them. With the concept of the life-world, however, Husserl embarked on a different path, which recognises that, even at its deepest level, consciousness is already embedded and operating in a world of meanings and pre-judgements that are socially, culturally and historically constituted. Phenomenology thereby became the study of consciousness and meaning in context (Dillon 2010).

The concepts, the life-world and intersubjectivity come from Alfred Schutz (1899–1959), who built on ideas from philosophers Husserl and Martin Heidegger (1889–1979) around the phenomenology of consciousness, meaning *the lived experience*, and Max Weber's idea of meaningful action. He emphasised the importance of the experience of the *life-world* as we experience it in everyday life with others as *intersubjectivity*. Schutz described how intersubjectivity created an apparently objective social world: 'the life world is an intersubjective world in which people both create social reality and are constrained by the preexisting social and cultural structures created by their predecessors' (Ritzer, 2011: 219). To see how intersubjectivity is relevant to nursing, consider Clare's story from the BBC Radio 4 play *Cancer Tales*, which features the experiences of a woman who has become a patient due to her cancer diagnosis: www.cancertales.org/elearning/home.html.

Scenario 1.3

Clare is a professional woman who is diagnosed with cancer of the uterus. Much of Clare's tale concerns issues around what makes a 'good doctor' in cancer care. In her view being a good doctor involves communicating diagnoses sensitively and effectively so that patients understand and can take the diagnosis 'in'; being a good doctor also involves continuity of care to patients – this is very important for Clare. Clare formulates this explicitly stating, 'what makes you into a good doctor is being humble, being able to learn from people'.

Clare's statement is an expression of her life-world – her experience of becoming a patient; the meaning she attaches to becoming a patient. Her life-world is and has been created in her interactions with her doctor as both of them construct intersubjective meaning to create social reality. This life-world shapes her understanding and experience of becoming a patient. Understanding how patients become patients, which includes their expectations of how doctors and nurses might act and behave, is integral to patients' life-worlds. That patients do create intersubjective meaning is central to patient-centred care, which we consider in the last section of this chapter.

Of course this approach to doctor–patient relationships is very different to Parsons' model which sees the doctor as active and the patient as passive.

We will now turn to Berger and Luckmann who studied the sociology of everyday life.

Sociology of everyday life

Sociologists such as Peter Berger (born 1929) and Thomas Luckmann (born 1927) were students of Schutz and were writing at the same time as Parsons but with very different viewpoints about social structures. They were interested in how social structures and processes were socially constructed, and how the individual exerted control over his social environment, his or her agency. Social structures for Berger and Luckmann were reproduced through individuals' actions; an ongoing or back-and-forth relationship between the individual and society produced and reproduced social structures. Their sociology studied the *reality of everyday life* and was concerned with intersubjectivity or the meanings that life had for individuals and small groups, the life-world. Here, then, are the links with phenomenology – a concern with the lived experience, the life-world and intersubjectivity.

Berger and Luckmann's work as well as Schutz's have not been used very much in nursing research which is surprising as their insights, in my view, have something to offer to nurses as they seek to understand patient experiences. Phenomenology more broadly has influenced a more recent development in sociological research into patient experience, narrative or story-telling, which we will consider now. Narrative in turn has also influenced an approach to care popular in the National Health Service (NHS) today, patient-centred care.

Narratives/patient experiences

Arthur Frank and Catherine Kohler Reissman, among others, have worked with patients' narratives – the stories patients tell to understand and explain their illnesses to themselves and to others at different points in time and to different audiences. These stories are ways of verbalising the life-world much as Clare does above. Kohler Reissman argues that a focus on patients' narratives redresses the medicalisation of illness and the ways in which the patient voice has been excluded from accounts of illness and with its focus on diagnosis and compliance. In other words, she argues that in accounts of the sick role, the patient's point of view has been excluded.

In another development, Mike Bury is a British sociologist whose work has focused on biographical disruption, how illness creates points at which individuals change identities and find new meaning, which is caused by the experience of both acute and chronic illness.

Reflection 1.6

Listen to Rita Charron's YouTube lecture – she talks about using patients' stories in her medical practice. It's a very different approach from Parsons. www.youtube.com/watch?v=24kHX2HtU3o.

She has used narrative in medical practice which is patient centred.

Another development in the UK has been the work of patient stories at the website Healthtalk.org which uses patients' stories to ensure their experiences are represented, voiced, understood and listened to.

Patient stories

Healthtalk.org comes from a unique partnership between a charity (DIPEx) and The Health Experiences Research Group (HERG) at the University of Oxford's Nuffield Department of Primary Care. The websites are managed by the charity and the research that appears on the sites is produced by the HERG team.

Healthtalk.org was created in 2001 by Oxford GP Dr Ann McPherson CBE and Dr Andrew Herxheimer after their own experiences of illness. Ann had been diagnosed with breast cancer and although she knew about the medical side, couldn't find anyone to talk to about what it was really like to have the disease. This, and Andrew's experience of knee-replacement surgery, prompted them to come up with the innovative idea of a patient-experience website.

A small group of people from various backgrounds formed a steering group and, after many meetings around Ann's kitchen table, the idea developed into the website that later became healthtalk.org (formerly Healthtalkonline and Youthhealthtalk). This is a powerful example of how patients (even when they are doctors) come together to challenge (resist) the status quo (the sick role). As Arthur Frank says, this resistance is the focus of micro sociology as a key theoretical approach in understanding how people become patients on their own terms.

Patient-centred care

So far we have considered the main sociological theories to explain the doctor–patient relationship or becoming a patient. The final section in this chapter is atheoretical; that is, it describes a perspective on being a patient that is not sociological but emerges from a sociological concern with patient agency and voice. Thus, we have considered the ways in which being a patient is constrained by social structures, shaped by the interactions between health professionals and patients, by subjectivity and personal meaning. We finish by considering how becoming a patient is constructed by patients themselves. This is as far removed from macro-sociological approaches as it is possible to be; it is a perspective that has merged from activism within sociology, health and feminism.

Patient-centred care has developed from sociological concerns with voice, inequality and agency (individuals being actively engaged in society). It is shaped by macro concerns with agency against structures and by micro concerns with voice and meaning.

Patient- or person-centred care is a framework for action to think about being a patient. It means that the hospital, health professional or community service must think about the service user, the patient, and have his or her needs at the forefront of service design and delivery. Simple enough you might say, but as we will see from the theories we discuss under macro sociology, it is sometimes difficult to abandon ways of thinking about patients when they have been dominant for a long time – actually roughly since the emergence of modern medicine.

Patient-centred care is the active involvement of patients and their families in the planning and delivery of care; sometimes it is referred to as new models of care.

It is endorsed by the National Institute for Clinical Excellence (NICE) in the UK (www.nice.org.uk/guidance/cg161/chapter/patient-centred-care) and reflected in the NHS Constitution (www.gov.uk/government/publications/the-nhs-constitution-for-england). It 'Provid[es] care that is respectful of and responsive to individual patient preferences, needs, and values, and ensuring that patient values guide all clinical decisions' (Wilkersen et al., 2010).

However, patient-centred care cannot mean anything unless there is active patient engagement in the design and evaluation of services. But how do we know what patients and their families want? Does every patient want to be actively engaged in decision-making in their own health, let alone in the design of health services and evaluating health-service delivery?

What do patients want?

Below is a link to a blog by Michael Seres who started posting his experience of small bowel transplant in 2011; Michael has Crohn's disease and surprisingly, given the amount of medication and surgery he has had, says he never felt like a patient until recently.

Reflection 1.7

Read Michael Seres' blog (http://beingapatient.blogspot.co.uk) to see what it's like to:

- live with a chronic, life-threatening disease;
- challenge the way doctors choose to interact with patients;
- involve family in care.

Having considered micro sociology, ask yourself what insights can be gained from this study of micro sociology, namely the study of the nuances of patient experience and the interactions between patients and the health professionals.

Michael Seres' blog is only one account of one patient's perspective of their illness and hospitalisation. As such it is not representative of others' experiences because we are all different. But we may share similar experiences and expectations. One way to find out how many patients experience being a patient is to ask lots of them using surveys.

Patient surveys

Patient surveys are one way to *measure* the quality of the service patients receive in patient surveys.

Reflection 1.8

Follow the link below and read Angela Coulter's short article 'Which patients get the worst deal?'

www.oecdobserver.org/news/archivestory.php/aid/560/Which_patients_get_the_worst_deal_.html

Then think about your responses to these questions:

- How is feedback from patients measured by the Picker Institute?
- Why do they measure patient feedback? Why not use patient stories?
- What problems are mentioned in the article as common to all countries surveyed?
- How would you explain the causes of these problems?

Even if we know a little about patients' experiences, is it all the responsibility of the health service or health professional? Do patients have responsibilities to behave in certain ways if treated as active partners in care, far from adopting the passive sick role, and to take responsibility for their health?

Patient responsibility

To some extent, it is now expected that patients are active, which is completely different from Parsons' sick-role theory.

Reflection 1.9

Watch the following videos for patients and see how being an active, knowledgeable patient is encouraged by GP Sarah Jarvis:

'Do you really need to see your GP?' (http://patient.info/health/media/videos/dr-sarah-jarvis-explains-do-i-really-need-to-see-my-gp)

'How to get the most out of seeing your GP' (http://patient.info/health/media/videos/dr-sarah-jarvis-says-how-to-make-the-most-of-gp-appointments).

Next time you are in your GP centre or in placement, have a look at the patient-condition leaflets written for patients. These are written for distribution nationally and on the website www.patient.co.uk/patientplus you will find advice under each disorder from public postings.

However, in the next chapter, we will consider the scale of health inequalities, including the social determinants of health. One of the social determinants is education and a question which might be asked about patient responsibility and patient information is: do all patients have the same access to being actively engaged? Don Berwick (2009), who is a strong advocate of patient-centred care, says it requires individuals to be informed. But not everyone has the means or education to become informed and, as we have seen, not all the health service is open and transparent. See Chapter 7 for further discussion of this point.

Chapter summary

In this chapter we have discussed sociological explanations of how people become patients. We have considered a model of understanding the doctor–patient relationship, Parsons' sick role, which was influential in medical sociology for over 30–40 years. We then thought about two sociological approaches to understanding the process of becoming a patient, symbolic interactionism and phenomenology, which contrasted with Parsons' model, before discussing narrative approaches where the voice of the patient is listened to above all else. Finally, we discussed patient-centred care, which is informed by the narrative and phenomenology.

In Chapter 2 we go on to think about who is a patient by exploring two important macro-sociological theories, Marxism and critical theory.

Going further

Arnstein, S. (1969) A ladder of citizen participation. *Journal of the American Institute of Planners* 35(4): 216–224.

Dillon, M. (2010) *Introduction to Sociological Theory: Theorists, Concepts and Their Applicability to the Twenty-First Century*. Chichester: Wiley-Blackwell.

Frank, A. (1995) *The Wounded Story Teller: Body, Illness and Ethics*. Chicago: University of Chicago Press.

Frank, A. (2014) From sick role to narrative subject: the sociological career of ill people and what's called 'experience'. Closing Plenary, British Sociological Association Medical Sociology Conference, Aston University, Birmingham. www.britsoc.co.uk/groups/bsa-medical-sociology/medsoc-video-archive.aspx

Goodman, B. (2013) Erving Goffman and the total institution. *Nurse Education Today* 33: 81–82. DOI: http://dx.doi.org/10.1016/j.nedt.2012.09.012.

Mitchell, E. (2013) The sick role. www.england.nhs.uk/2013/09/30/ed-mitchell-2/.

Strauss, A.L. (1975) *Chronic Illness and the Quality of Life*. St. Louis: Mosby.

See this website for a student nurse's take on Parsons' role theory: http://mentalhealthnurse-training.wordpress.com/2012/11/03/functionalism-and-the-sick-role-sociology-and-mental-health-nursing/.

Try watching this video on YouTube to understand a little more of what structural functionalism is about: www.youtube.com/watch?v=mpDVs3Uifjg.

Look at these YouTube clips for more about Parsons: www.youtube.com/watch?v=gJT1oHqlFis

Have a look at Ed Mitchell's brief description of Parsons' role theory and how long-term conditions have changed our understanding of the sick role www.england.nhs.uk/2013/09/30/ed-mitchell-2/

Essay on Parsons' role theory and operating theatres: http://usir.salford.ac.uk/2753/5/Sick_Role_JAN_FINAL.pdf.

Varul's paper on role theory and chronic illness: http://bod.sagepub.com.ezproxy.mdx.ac.uk/content/16/2/72.full.pdf+html.

Burnham on why sociologists abandoned the sick-role concept: http://hhs.sagepub.com.ezproxy.mdx.ac.uk/content/27/1/70.full.pdf+html.

Read more about patients' stories:

www.healthtalk.org/about/overview
www.healthtalk.org/peoples-experiences
www.healthtalk.org/peoples-experiences/mental-health
www.kevinmd.com/blog/2011/08/patient-unforgettable-form-medical-education.html

References

Allan, H.T. (2002) Nursing the clinic, being there, hovering: ways of caring in a British fertility unit. *Journal of Advanced Nursing* 38(1): 86–93.

Allan, H.T. and Barber, D. (2005) Emotion boundary work in advanced fertility nursing roles. *Nursing Ethics* 12(4): 391–400.

Berwick, D. (2009) What 'patient-centered' should mean: confessions of an extremist. *Health Affairs* 28(4): 555–565.

Blumer, H. (1962) Society as symbolic interaction. In A.M. Rose (ed.) *Human Behaviour and Social Processes*. Boston, MA: Houghton Mifflin.

Bone, M. et al. (1992) *Retirement and Retirement Plans*. London: HMSO.

Chamberlain-Salaun, J., Mills, J. and Usher, K. (2013) Linking symbolic interactionism and grounded theory methods in a research design: from Corbin & Strauss's assumptions to actions. SageOpen DOI:10.1177/2158244013505757.

Dillon, M. (2010) *Introduction to Sociological Theory: Theorists, Concepts and Their Applicability to the Twenty-First Century*. Chichester: Wiley-Blackwell.

Frank, A. (2014) BSA Medical Sociology Annual Conference 2014 Closing Plenary: Professor Arthur Frank. https://vimeo.com/109902249.

Garmarnikov, E. (1978) Sexual division of labour: the case of nursing. In A. Kuhn and A. Wolpe (eds) *Feminism and Materialism*. London: Routledge & Kegan Paul, pp. 96–123.

Glaser B.G. and Strauss, A. (1964) *Awareness of Dying*. Chicago: Aldine.

Glaser B.G. and Strauss, A. (1968) *A Time for Dying*. Chicago: Aldine.

Goodman, B. (2013) Erving Goffman and the total institution. *Nurse Education Today* 33: 81–82.

Henderson, A. (2006) Boundaries around the 'well-informed' patient: the contribution of Schutz to inform nurses' interactions. *Journal of Clinical Nursing* 15 (1): 4–10.

Lo, S.F., Hu, W.Y., Hayter, M., Chang, S.C., Hsu, M.Y. and Wu, L.Y. (2008) Experience of living with a malignant fungating wound: a qualitative study. *Journal of Clinical Nursing* 17(20) 2699–2708.

Overgaard, S. and Zahavi, D. (2007) Phenomenological sociology: the subjectivity of everyday life. Available at: http://cfs.ku.dk/staff/zahavi-publications/sociology.pdf.

Parsons, T. (1951) *The Social System*. Glencoe, IL: Free Press.

Parsons, T. (1975) The sick role and the role of the physician reconsidered. *Milbank Memorial Fund Quarterly/Health and Society* 53: 257–78.

Revans, R.W. (1964) *Standards for Morale: Cause and Effect in Hospitals*. Published for the Nuffield Provincial Hospitals Trust. London: Oxford University Press

Ritzer, G. (2011) *Sociological Theory*. New York: McGraw Hill.

Roger, A., Pilgrim, D. and Lacey, R (1993) *Experiencing Psychiatry: Users' Views of Services*. Basingstoke: Macmillan.

Scheff, T.J. (1974) The labelling theory of mental illness. *American Sociological Review* 39(3): 444–452.

Schon, D. (1983) *The Reflective Practitioner: How Professionals Think in Action*. New York: Basic Books

Sewell, H. (2009) *Working with Ethnicity, Race and Culture in Mental Health: A Handbook for Practitioners*. London: Jessica Kingsley.

Strauss, A., Fagerhaugh, S., Suczek, B. and Wiener, C. (1982) Sentimental work in the technologised hospital. *Sociology of Health & Illness* 4(3): 254–278.

Varul, M.T. (2010) Talcott Parsons, the sick role and chronic illness. *Body & Society* 16(2): 72–94.

Wilkerson, V., Fung, C.-C., May, W. and Elliott, D. (2010) Assessing patient-centered care: one approach to health disparities education. *Journal of General Internal Medicine* V25(Supp. 2): 86–90.

Wilkinson, G. (1999) *Power and Nursing Practice*. Basingstoke: Macmillan.

Willems, S., de Maesschalck, S., Deveugele, M. and Derese, A. (2005) Socio-economic status of the patient and doctor–patient communication: does it make a difference? *Journal of Patient Education Counselling* 56(2): 139–146.

Winterbourne View Hospital (2012) *Final Report*. London: Department of Health. Available at: www.gov.uk/government/uploads/system/uploads/attachment_data/file/213215/final-report.pdf.

2

Who is the patient?

Helen Allan

In Chapter 1 we thought about how people became patients, how the doctor–patient relationship might be described and how sociologists have moved in their understanding of the patient experience from Parsons' sick role to Arthur Frank's narrative of patient experience. We moved essentially from sociological theory which understood the world from a macro perspective to one in which the micro side of social life was more important. Often it is a balance or interaction between the two.

The issue

In a recent seminar, I was showing a class of first-year student nurses a video clip that dealt with health inequalities. The video followed a family who lived on social benefits and did not have much spare money. The group were divided by their views on how the family should spend their benefits.

Some students thought that the family were unable to make 'healthy' eating choices because of 'poor' spending decisions in other areas, such having a satellite dish and a huge TV. Indeed, there appeared to be no main meal of the day for these children.

Other students felt the family should be entitled to spend their money as they wished and that freedom gave them autonomy, which was more important than healthy eating.

Imagine you were these children's health visitor. What are the issues you would discuss with your team in respect of these children's access to healthy eating and, more broadly, healthy lifestyles?

In this chapter we consider the topic of life chances and health inequalities from three sociological perspectives (see below). The reason this is an issue is because in the UK there are quite glaring health inequalities which you as student nurses ought to a) be aware of, b) understand how and why they exist, and c) begin to see how nursing might address inequalities in practice – this is extremely difficult and we certainly don't expect you to singlehandedly resolve them but we signpost you to some examples of where nurses have worked to reduce health inequalities.

Chapter outline

The chapter is divided into three broad sections:

- How the political economy of health shapes who is a patient – social class inequalities
- Gender, race/ethnicity, age and the social reproduction of health inequalities
- Medicalisation, patient empowerment and emancipatory knowledge

We are about to consider a very different view to Parsons, and indeed symbolic interactionists and phenomenologists, around the experience of becoming a patient. These perspectives argue that society might actually be causing your illness.

The political economy of health and how it shapes being a patient in a capitalist health system

The idea that society makes us ill is grounded in ideas around political economy that were first articulated by Karl Marx in the nineteenth century. Marx didn't write about health in the focused way as Parsons so we have to delve a bit into sociological theory and the history of capitalism to understand how Marxism explains illness and being a patient.

The founding fathers of sociology

Marx, along with Emile Durkheim and Max Weber, are known as the founding fathers of sociology as they established the discipline in the mid- to late-nineteenth century. They also had rather good beards. Go to the website in the box below for an overview of sociology and the founding fathers – and check out the beards.

Reflection 2.1 (on beards)

http://blogs.exeter.ac.uk/unfinishedbusiness/blog/2013/10/05/sociology-and-the-bearded-bourgeois-white-men/

The emergence of capitalism

Marx was writing at a time when capitalism as an economic system, a way of organising the production of goods, had emerged in Western Europe as the dominant form of social organisation. Capitalism has been adopted virtually globally and brings us many benefits, as Marx himself acknowledged. I'd far rather be a nurse living in 2015 than a peasant living in a feudal society with no freedom of movement and a life expectancy of 35/40 years of age! However, as Marx also argued, capitalism has extensive downsides, especially if you are not wealthy or educated or living in the West.

Another less appealing feature of the emergence of capitalism is its association – particularly in the UK – with the slave trade and colonisation. Have a look at this website for a short overview of the links between capitalism and slavery: http://revealinghistories.org.uk/how-did-money-from-slavery-help-develop-greater-manchester/articles/the-rise-of-capitalism-and-the-development-of-europe.html.

Capitalism is a mode or way of producing goods – whether those are luxury goods or food – where the means of production (producing) are privately owned by individuals, families or corporations (we'd probably say shareholders nowadays). Marx considered anyone who owned private wealth as part of the *bourgeoisie*. So, the *bourgeoisie* as a class benefit from the production of goods. The factory owner owns the factory or the farmer owns the farm and both benefit from any wealth created by the sale of the goods produced; that is, they own the means of production. But how much they sell is dependent on the productivity of the workers who actually produce the goods to sell. In this system, the workers or *proletariat* sell their labour, that is their ability to work, in order to live. Of course, we may not think of ourselves as labourers if we work as health professionals, but if we don't own the means of production, that, according to Marx, is what we are. This disparity in wealth brought about by ownership or non-ownership of the means of production, private ownership, creates class relations that are often antagonistic and unequal. This is important and we shall come back to it later in this chapter when we consider health inequalities which are ultimately based on class inequalities and wealth or the lack thereof.

Social relations of production

Marx was writing at a time when Europe was experiencing social revolution. The French Revolution (1789–1799) was the first period of immense social upheaval in Europe, followed by revolutions in (again) France, Germany, Italy and Austria in 1848 – think *Les Misérables*. These were attempts to subvert the social order, to protest against the owners of the means of production. The times in which Marx wrote are important because his view is that societies are moving towards a state of communism where there is no social inequality and where all own the means of production; that is, all work for the good of everyone and not for individual profit. It was the ownership of the means of production, where a bourgeois owned his factory, employed workers and exploited them to extract maximum profit, which he wanted to change. Marx called the relationships between workers and owners of the means of production the *relations of production* or individuals' social position vis-à-vis private ownership and labour.

Reflection 2.2

We introduced the idea of social class inequalities in Chapter 1. Now have a look at the following statistics.

Within the UK, the top 10 per cent of the population is now 100 times as wealthy as the bottom 10 per cent. As far as income is concerned, in 2010 chief executives' pay in successful companies was 145 times the average salary for workers, and it is on track to be 214 times the average salary by 2020 (www.cost_ofliving.net). These inequalities seem to be increasing after diminishing during the post-Second World War period.

Why do you think these inequalities are a) so stark and b) so entrenched?

If Marx's analysis seems far removed from the twenty-first century, remember that Marx and Charles Dickens both wrote about exploitative factory conditions at roughly the same time. Read *Oliver Twist* by Dickens and then think of factory conditions for workers in the garment industry in India and the scandals that emerge from time to time about loss of life as factories, built to maximise profit, collapse because they are unsafe.

You might think that such exploitative conditions at work are something to do with the past. Have a look at Graham Scambler's blog at www.discoversociety. org/2013/12/03/from-power-elite-to-governing-oligarchy/ for a short analysis of current wealth inequalities between rich and poor in the UK.

Such conditions affect workers in the health services too as Bolton and Wibberley's (2014) research shows.

Reflection 2.3

Consider Bolton and Wibberley's paper (2014), which focuses on the exploitative working conditions of domiciliary carers; their work conditions are constrained by the employers' needs to keep costs down to meet the commissioners' contracts demands.

Bolton and Wibberley give the example of the employers booking each home visit so that as one finishes another starts leaving no time for travel. But worse, travel time is not paid for either – by the commissioners or by the employers. The carers Bolton and Wibberley describe are certainly disempowered through the relations of production in their work and the owners of the care companies profit from what is a form of market economy. But the situation is complex as the commissioners, sitting on clinical commissioning groups, also profit by paying less for care. Of course these commissioners represent us, the tax payers, and the state. And ironically these same taxpayers, that is the patients who receive care, have less and less time with their carers. It is not a simple market economy that is the context here (unlike, for example, farming and price setting in terms of milk production) but a contractual system not necessarily based on a supply–demand relationship.

We will now consider Marx's explanations for these conditions.

Base and superstructure

For Marx, capitalism was an economic form that determined society. He called this the base and superstructure model. The base of society is the economy and this determines other societal structures such as education, religion and family life.

These relations of production constitute the economic structure of society, the real foundation, on which rises a legal and political superstructure and to which correspond definite forms of social consciousness ... social, political and intellectual life processes in general. It is not the consciousness of men that determines their existence, but their social existence that determines their consciousness. (Marx, 1859: 80)

This was revolutionary because Marx was saying that society is shaped by the economy; and at the time, and even now, this meant he viewed society differently to how it had been viewed. It wasn't the natural order of things, it couldn't be explained by religious belief; it was socially constructed by men (and women – although they didn't feature much in Marx's writing) themselves. So if you were poor, you didn't have to be content with your lot; you could work with others to change your social situation. And for social existence, read economy, and then, as now, capitalism. Indeed religious belief, specifically the Methodist movement in the nineteenth century, was described by Marx as the 'opium of the people' – believers were told 'don't drink, don't gamble, work hard and accept your lot here on earth – you will be rewarded in heaven'.

We forget that our health system is determined by capitalism. In the UK it is more acceptable perhaps to talk of 'privatisation', forgetting that introducing private capital into the provision of health services means opening up new markets to private capital and capitalists.

Reflection 2.4

Think of recent debates about the privatisation of the National Health Service (NHS): www.bbc.co.uk/news/health-28581878.

Ask yourself what are the advantages and for whom of a privatised health service.

Then ask yourself what are the advantages of a publically funded health service and for whom.

In this chapter we consider to some extent the degree to which the drug industry (a commercial capitalist enterprise) shapes healthcare.

Social class today

Marx was writing over 160 years ago. So are social class and the social relations of production still relevant to student nurses, indeed ourselves as British citizens, today? Some sociologists think so. According to the previously mentioned blog by Graham Scambler, power and wealth are now more concentrated than ever, possibly even more so than in Marx's day. Scambler argues that an oligarchy or super rich class now control this concentrated wealth, and that class, shaped by capitalist relations of production, determines our social positions.

But Scambler, an eminent medical sociologist (1951–), helpfully points out that social class isn't quite what it was 50 years ago; we no longer *feel* as constrained by our class position as our parents or our grandparents used to. He calls this the subjective nature of social class. But the objective class positions of the wealthy 1 per cent of the population vis-à-vis the rest of population, irrespective of whether they are working or middle class, are nevertheless real and unequal.

So how is social class measured? Traditionally in the UK we've used the five-class scheme Registrar General's Social Class (RGSC), which was created in 1911 and a variation of this scheme was still used until recently. In 2001, the National Statistics Socio-Economic Classification (NS-SEC) replaced the RGSC. For a description of the new scheme see www.statistics.gov.uk. And for a comparison of both see Table 2.1.

We might accept Scambler's suggestion that social class is more subjective now than it was when Marx was writing, and that individuals might feel less identification with these categories. Nevertheless, there are identifiable differences if we use social class as an indicator between individuals' income and social positioning, that is spending power, consumption and even educational achievement.

There are also sharp differences between how wealth is distributed across households in the UK. Figure 2.1 illustrates this inequality using wealth distribution by total number of households divided into fifths.

Table 2.1   Classifications of social classes

RGSC	NS-SEC	Typical class occupation
I Professional occupations	I Senior professionals/ senior managers	Corporate managers, corporate administrative roles, doctors, university lecturers
II Managerial and technical occupations	II Associate professionals/ junior managers	Journalists, nurses, teachers, science, business, media professionals
III Skilled occupations manual (M) and non-manual (N)	III Other administrative and clerical workers	Police (sergeant and below), armed services, travel agents
	IV Own account non-professional	Farmers, taxi drivers, hotel managers
IV Partly skilled occupations	V Supervisors, technicians and related workers	Train drivers, electricians, bakers
	VI Intermediate workers	Sales, administrative, secretarial or related, traffic wardens, dental nurses
V Unskilled occupations	VII Other workers	Building labourers, farmworkers, cleaners, waiters
	VIII Never worked/other inactive	Never worked, long-term unemployed, students

© Crown copyright 2015. Adapted from data from the Office for National Statistics licensed under the Open Government Licence v.3.0

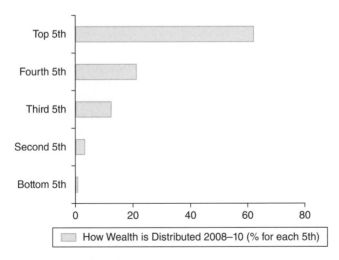

Figure 2.1   Wealth and Assets Survey, Wave 2 Birmingham Wealth Commission (total wealth including private pension rights)

(http://discoversociety.org/2013/12/03/focus-the-distribution-of-wealth-what-we-think-and-how-it-is/)

Adapted from data from the University of Birmingham Wealth Commission, reproduced with permission from Karen Rowlingson

The implications of these data and the theory of social class are that being unemployed, or in a social class where your income is low, means that you and your family will be less wealthy and, importantly, have less healthy lives. You will be less likely to go to the doctor to report signs of ill health, work in occupations that make you sicker, attend less frequently for preventative healthcare, have less money to eat healthily. And you won't have access to informal networks that support you when you are ill or access to shops where fresh food is sold. This sounds far-fetched but as Tudor Hart argued, 'The availability of good medical care tends to vary inversely with the need for it in the population served' (1971: 405). This medical care applies to the provision of transport, shops with fresh food; chemists; every sort of service that one needs to maintain a healthy life.

Reflection 2.5

For greater understanding of these issues and in particular how being poor as a child affects your life chances, have a look at these two sources and then reconsider our issue at the beginning of this chapter and ask whether your answers to the questions you were asked would be the same now having read this chapter so far.

See this link to the *Guardian*: www.theguardian.com/commentisfree/2013/may/08/rising-child-poverty-uk-poorer.

Search the Child Poverty Action Group website: www.cpag.org.uk/child-poverty-facts-and-figures.

Finally, even when visiting the doctor, working-class patients may be treated differently from middle-class patients, probably because they don't share what Bourdieu calls *habitus* or the same social understandings, accent, ways of explaining yourself, dress and so on. All these social processes result in social and health inequalities.

For a more detailed reading of the debates around social class, see Michelle Dillon's *Introduction to Sociological Theory* or Anthony Giddens and Phillip Suttons' *Sociology*.

The social determinants of health and illness

The phrase 'It is not the consciousness of men that determines their existence, but their social existence that determines their consciousness' is central to our application of Marxist ideas to health and to why some sociologists talk about the political economy of health (Porter, 1998). Marx was arguing that the economic base on which society is organised, the nature of capitalism which is based on unequal distribution of social resources, exposes workers to poorer health than the wealthy in society, namely those who own the means of production. In other words, health is determined by class which is itself determined by the economy.

So why is social class and wealth important when considering how individuals become patients?

Reflection 2.6

Have a look at the following YouTube video clip 'Health Inequalities – Social Determinants of Health Film': www.youtube.com/watch?v=aS3-MZZyVNI.

The social determinants of health include: education, housing, transport, access to shops, street lighting, the built environment and financial security (employment). See Figure 2.2 which shows Dahlgren and Whitehead's rainbow model of the social determinants of health. As you will see from this model, these social factors interact with other factors such as age, sex and hereditary (biological) conditions and predispositions, as well as family and community-level social networks.

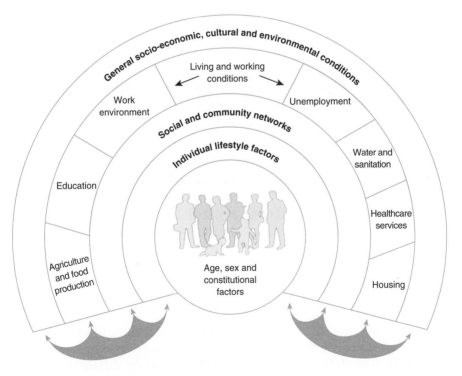

Figure 2.2 The main determinants of health

Source: Dahlgren and Whitehead (1993).

Health inequalities

Health inequalities are differences in health status or in the distribution of health determinants between different population groups, that is men, women, children, in social class I compared to those in social class V.

There have been health inequalities since the beginning of the NHS and, of course, long before. One important report into health inequalities, the Black Report from 1980, showed that the death rate for men in social class V was twice that for men in social class I and that the gap between the two was increasing rather than reducing, as was expected with the introduction of the NHS. (NHSE have a good concise history of the Black report along with a potted history of the NHS at: www.nhs.uk/NHSEngland/thenhs/nhshistory/Pages/NHShistory1980s.aspx.)

The most recent statistics on health inequalities include:

- Unskilled workers are twice as likely to die of cancer as professionals.
- There is an 18.5-year difference in good health years that men in Scotland will live between the least and most deprived areas.
- In England people living in the most deprived areas will die seven years, in Northern Ireland eight years and in Scotland 11 years before those living in the wealthiest areas (ONS, 2014).

Reflection 2.7

Watch this Andrew Marr YouTube video on life expectancy and think about how life expectancy is affected by your social circumstances and factors such as diet. www.youtube.com/watch?v=KvwIW2dlUj8

These statistics are repeated at the level of individual illness and condition across the life span and across geographic location measured by local authority, parish and other government boundaries.

But why is all this important? Because who you are, where you live and what resources you have to draw on when ill affect your recovery but also your overall life chances.

Scenario 2.1

Imagine you are working on a medical ward where there are patients recovering from a heart attack (myocardial infarction). You have been asked by your mentor to read the information on lifestyle choices that the ward staff give out to patients on recovery post-infarction. Yet it says nothing about class inequalities.

Can you think of an argument to convince your mentor to include some-thing that reflects class inequalities, knowing as you do that: a solicitor who can join a gym, buy low-carb, low-fat, fresh foods at Waitrose and reduce their hours at work will be far more likely to follow the ward advice than a single mum of three children who works as a cleaner and lives in the least desirable area of town with poor access to fresh foods and no free income to join a gym.

So what should your mentor do when presented with this information?

How does undertanding social class inform our everyday practice as a nurse?

Despite these arguments and statistics being (for me at least) convincing evidence that social and health inequalities persist in the UK today, can this be explained only by social class, as Marx argued?

What neither Marx nor Weber considered were inequalities based on gender, race/ethnicity and age. So how do gender, race/ethnicity and age shape being a patient?

Gender, race/ethnicity, age and the social reproduction of health inequalities

Being a patient is therefore shaped or constrained by the social class you might belong to; but it is also shaped or constrained by your gender, race/ethnicity and age.

Gender

'Women get sick and men die.' This fact has held constant since childbirth became safer for women (since the Second World War), but the advantage women have over men in terms of living longer is decreasing. How do women's mortality rates compare to men's recently and about 50 years ago?

In 1963, male mortality rates at all ages were higher than those for females. In 2013, infant mortality rates remain slightly higher for males, with 4.4 deaths per 1,000 live births compared with 3.5 for females. Mortality rates in 2013 for ages 1 to 4, 5 to 9, and 10 to 14 years were the same for both sexes, whilst male rates were higher for those aged 15 years and over. So a shift is beginning very slowly early on in life.

Reflection 2.8

One statistic that has remained stubbornly persistent over the years is that men commit suicide more than women. What reasons can you think of?

You should watch this video clip which provides some answers: https://www.youtube.com/watch?v=68v5-inOdao.

What of later in life?

At older ages the relative difference in mortality between males and females is more notable. In 1963, at ages 55 to 69, male mortality rates were double those for females. By 2013, the relative difference in mortality for these ages had reduced, with mortality rates around 1.5 times higher for males than females. The absolute difference in mortality at these ages also reduced by more than half over the same period.

However, this still means that in 2012 women had 82.6 years and men 78.7 years life expectancy. Even at age 65, women are expected to live 20.7 years and men 18.2 years.

These figures measure mortality but what if we look at years lived without disability, or disability-free life expectancy (DFLE)?

We can measure DFLE between a wealthier local authority (West Sussex) compared with a poorer local authority (County Durham) to show how social class interacts with gender (see Figure 2.3). So West Sussex in the South East of England has almost twice the wealth per household as the North East of England and the advantage in mortality of females over males increases at age 65 in terms of DFLE. In County Durham, which is poorer in terms of wealth per household, the advantage is less at birth compared with West Sussex and decreases over time.

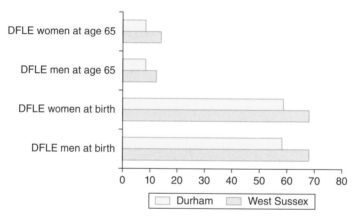

Figure 2.3   DFLE in men and women at birth and at age 65 compared between West Sussex and Durham

Source: www.equalitytrust.org.uk/about-inequality/scale-and-trends/scale-economic-inequality-uk.

The Office for National Statistics explains the gradual narrowing of the gender health inequalities gap by saying:

> The general narrowing of the gap between male and female mortality rates can be explained by a number of reasons including improvements in male health leading to a rise in male life expectancy which has increased at a greater rate than for females. (National Life Tables, 2011–13)

Increases in women entering the labour force over the last 50 years are considered to have had an impact on levels of stress, smoking and drinking, leading to changes in the health of females (ONS, 2011, 2013; Steptoe et al., 1998). So it may be bad news for women that our social lives are less healthy than our mothers' or grand-mothers' but consider the following: 22 per cent of men in England and Wales die before the age of 65 (compared to 13 per cent of women); and 42 per cent die before 75 (compared to 26 per cent of women); 76 per cent of people who kill themselves are men; and men are 70 per cent more likely to die from a cancer that affects both men and women.

Irrespective of improving health for men, women still have a mortality advantage. So how are these differences explained? Partly through social class and partly through gender. Biologists argue it's biology or evolution; while sociologists argue it's more our lifestyle interacting with social behaviours that are socially constrain-ing. For example, women are 'used' to more surveillance of their bodies during menarche, pregnancy and menopause so perhaps it's no surprise that they attend doctors more for health prevention at other times of their lives. Men still smoke more than women and still have more dangerous occupations.

Reflection 2.9

Consider your group of friends or perhaps fellow students. What reasons can you give to explain their healthy and unhealthy behaviours? How far is this determined by gender, social class or education?

Or does being a student diminish those gender and class differences?

Consider what sort of advice you could develop to change unhealthy behaviours in students. Which would be more amenable to change and which would be difficult?

What conclusions can you draw about the effects on health of a) gender, b) social class, c) peer groups?

Race/ethnicity

Race and ethnicity are further social factors that determine health in our unequal society. For example, Public Health England states that the infant mortality rate in England varies substantially by ethnic group (www.lho.org.uk/LHO_Topics/National_Lead_Areas/HealthInequalitiesOverview.aspx):

> In 2005–06, the infant mortality rate among the Black groups (8.0 deaths per 1,000 live births), as well as the Asian groups (6.9 deaths per 1,000 live births), was significantly higher than that of the White ethnic groups (4.4 deaths per 1,000 live births).

Unfortunately, later in life, these figures don't get any better when we consider risk-taking behaviour such as smoking:

- Bangladeshi men were 43 per cent more likely (risk ratio of 1.43) and Irish men were 30 per cent more likely (risk ratio of 1.30) to smoke cigarettes than the general male population after accounting for age. Indian men were less likely (risk ratio of 0.78) to smoke cigarettes than the general male population in England.

- Smoking is less common among women in most – but not all – minority ethnic groups compared with the general female population, when age is taken into account. Compared with the general female population, Bangladeshi women were the least likely to smoke cigarettes (risk ratio of 0.11), followed by Pakistani women (risk ratio of 0.19), Indian women (risk ratio of 0.23), Chinese women (risk ratio of 0.32) and black African women (risk ratio 0.34). However, Irish and black Caribbean women were as likely to report cigarette smoking as the general population for women.

Unfortunately, while smoking may be reduced in some ethnic groups, chewing tobacco isn't and gives rise to higher rates of oropharyngeal cancer.

Differences between different ethnic populations are also evident when looking at chronic disease in the UK.

Type 2 diabetes accounts for at least 90% of diabetes worldwide. The prevalence among the white European population varies from 2% overall to 10% in [the] age group above 70 years. It is much more common in the ethnic minorities groups residing in the developed countries; South Asian and African-Caribbean groups in the UK in particular have a high prevalence. . . .

The prevalence of adult type 2 diabetes is about three to five times greater in African-Caribbean and South Asian people respectively compared with the white European population. The prevalence of diabetes is not substantially different among Chinese compared with the general UK population. (Oldroyd et al., 2005: 486–487)

Reflection 2.10

Consider the fact: You are more likely to develop type 2 diabetes if you are from an Afro-Caribbean or South Asian community than if you are white European by three to five times. See Oldroyd et al. (2005).

Oldroyd and his colleagues don't just point out these alarming facts but consider how health services might tackle prevention and treatment in different ethnic groups to address these inequalities. They discuss how interacting factors, the social and biological determinants of health, all play their part in explaining these differences between ethnic groups living in the UK. They also point out that determining ethnicity is hugely difficult when studying disease at population level and makes our understanding of these interacting factors complicated.

Collecting social data on the basis of race and/or ethnicity is problematic. Race was traditionally considered to be the individual or group's biological characteristics such as hair type, eye and skin colour; ethnicity referred to the social or cultural factors such as language, cultural symbols and practices such as eating and drinking, although it could also refer to nation, a sense of belonging and religion.

This is clearly seen in the following UNESCO statement made in 1950:

National, religious, geographic, linguistic and cultural groups do not necessarily coincide with racial groups: and the cultural traits of such groups have no demonstrated genetic connection with racial traits. Because serious errors of this kind are habitually committed when the term 'race' is used in popular parlance, it would be better when speaking of human races to drop the term 'race' altogether and speak of 'ethnic groups'. (The Race Question: http://unesdoc.unesco.org/images/0012/001282/128291eo.pdf)

And in the next statement, anthropologist David Griffith makes clear the link between capitalism, colonialism and the concept of race:

The opposing interests that divide the working classes are further reinforced through appeals to "racial" and "ethnic" distinctions. Such appeals serve to allocate different categories of workers to rungs on the scale of labor markets, relegating stigmatized populations to the lower levels and insulating the higher echelons from competition from below. Capitalism did not create all the distinctions of ethnicity and race that function to set off categories of workers from one another. It is, nevertheless, the process of labor mobilization under capitalism that imparts to these distinctions their effective values. (1987:840)

In addition, ethnicity is a subjective category. Consider what happens when you fill in the Census question about your ethnic background; you choose, so it's subjective. Therefore any data may be based on subjective judgements not objective facts.

Age

Eighty per cent of all deaths in England and Wales occur in people over age 65. Two-thirds of people with limited long-term illness or disability are aged 55 and over. Yet most research into health inequalities focuses on the younger age groups (Grundy and Holt, 2005).

In addition, there are differences between those aged 55–74 and those aged over 75–84 years of age that are the consequence of life events and experiences of deprivation. Grundy and Holt (2005: 5) explain these differences by relative wealth over a life span: 'those who [follow] more disadvantaged pathways through their adult lives, as marked out by longer periods of employment, earlier age at marriage and more children, were at greater risk of reporting ill-health and illness'.

Reflection 2.11

Have a look at this video which addresses the difference in age death rates: www.youtube.com/watch?v=r0cJ7CX1lCA.

What explanations are given in the video for these differences in age ratios?

What additional explanations can you think of from your experience of caring for older people so far in your nurse training?

How far might age, race/ethnicity and gender interact in explaining these age differences?

So, in other words, social deprivation, as Grundy and Holt say, over a lifetime and over a range of measures of social deprivation (education attainment, car owner- ship, income, housing ownership and household resources), result in poorer health outcomes for social classes IV and V than social classes I, II and III (www.lancaster. ac.uk/fass/projects/hvp/pdf/nl7art2.pdf).

Interestingly, Grundy and Holt also used biological determinants such as height as well as social indicators such as education. Lack of stature and education were associated with poorer health in both older age groups 65–74 and 75–84.

Further analyses of social support and poor health in the 75–84 age group showed that poor health was highest among the divorced men and lowest in married men. In women, it was the opposite: poor health was lowest among single women and highest among married women. Across all social classes, those reporting poor health were more likely to lack social support. This is similar to other work by Sara Arber (2013).

So far we have argued that being a patient is shaped by our family background and our social circumstances including access to wealth. Our health both in real time and in the future as elderly people is shaped by our social class position, who our parents were and what we do in terms of employment, but more than that: what our educational achievement is, where we live, what type of housing we live in, our diet and transport.

In the last section on macro approaches to *being a patient*, we will consider work by writers from the Frankfurt School in Germany in the 1920–1930s who included Adorno, Horkheimer, Marcuse and Pollock. Their work is collectively called critical theory and there were two strands: literary theory (not our concern here) and sociol- ogy which built on Marx's writings (among others). Their work is so varied that we don't have time to cover it here in any depth but a good introduction is Sam Porter's book *Social Theory and Nursing Practice* (1998).

Medicalisation, patient empowerment and emancipatory knowledge

Critical theorists considered that our health was determined, rather than merely shaped, by our social class. They used Marxist ideas about the nature of capitalism and how it structures social classes according to their wealth and ownership of the means of production to understand how even the knowledge produced in academia is fundamentally produced (mostly indirectly) by capitalism for the benefit of the wealthy (the bourgeoisie) at the expense of the poor (working classes). So an example might be the pharmaceutical industry which invests in research from which it foresees a return in the future. The Director-General of the World Health Organization recently caused a stir by saying that the pharmaceutical industry 'has no incentive to develop drugs for poor countries which can't pay' (4 November 2014: http://time. com/3555706/who-ebola-vaccine-pharmaceutical-industry-margaret-chan/).

What the Director-General said is that the pharmaceutical industry develops drugs that are profitable and, as the Ebola epidemic in 2014 showed, has failed to develop a drug to combat Ebola because it is a disease of poor countries who would not be able to pay for the cost of any new drug: 'The R&D incentive is virtually nonexistent', she continued, 'A profit-driven industry does not invest in products for markets that cannot pay'. So knowledge is not value free but developed through research which is funded by capitalist enterprises. This is what critical theorists pointed out: that knowledge as well as social structures are shaped by class relations and the ownership of the means of production, that is, wealth.

Busfield (2010) and Tiggle (2007) both talk about how medicine and the pharmaceutical industry have joined forces to produce a dependence on drugs in modern society. Their model of the doctor's role is very different to Parsons as they argue that doctors' practice is shaped by the pharmaceutical industry and endorsed, if not encouraged, by government, sometimes to the detriment of the patient.

The Ebola example and the papers by Busfield and Tiggle certainly make it clear that class relations are oppressive both nationally and globally. We have seen how a Marxist view of society assumes that the control of material resources through class position (Porter, 1998) is oppressive for those denied access to wealth, and results in social inequalities. And material resources include education and housing as well as capital or wealth. We have also illustrated the clear links between class position and health and illness, or health inequalities. Oppression can also arise in social relations between social classes and ethnic groups. Critical theorists echo Marxist concerns with oppression and add another level of oppression, dominant forms of knowledge which obscure subordinate forms of knowledge through oppressive social structures (Porter, 1998) such as academia, publishing and professional accreditation.

Scenarios 2.2 and 2.3

By dominant and subordinate forms of knowledge we mean that certain forms of knowledge are valued more than others; subordinate knowledge may even be ridiculed by people who claim to know better than others. You might have had some experience of this in your time as a student nurse.

An example might be a patient who has a long-term chronic illness and feels his or her knowledge of their own condition is not listened to by their doctor. The patient struggles to assert their point of view.

Or take this example:

A patient is critically ill in intensive care, on life-support. His condition is so unstable that the medical team direct the nurses not to wash him, turn him or do any mouth care. The nurses disagree with this as they feel his comfort is still a priority even when his condition is unstable and when the long-term outcome is poor. However, the medical team argue that the empirical knowledge they have of his vital signs outweigh the ethical and aesthetic knowledge the nurses cite. His condition continues to deteriorate and the doctors agree in his final days for the patient to have nursing care.

In this example, the dominant knowledge is the empirical pathophysiological knowledge and the subordinate knowledge is the nursing knowledge which is based on aesthetics and ethics (Carper, 1979).

Emancipation and empowerment

In Marx's writings and in the writings of the Frankfurt School we find a concern with empowerment and emancipation. Consider the second example above, and how the nurses struggled to argue that their knowledge is as valued as the empirical knowledge. Or the first example, where the patient with the long-term illness might suggest that their subjective feelings and symptoms are equally as important to the overall medical management as the signs their doctor observes. They are both examples of using emancipatory actions against the power of the doctor.

Nurse education in the 1980s was influenced by these ideas and a concern with empowerment and emancipatory action is embedded in nursing education curricula through reflection which forms part of your learning.

Empowerment and emancipation are core concepts in education and health today and are also represented in the NHS Constitution (www.nhs.uk/NHSEngland/thenhs/about/Pages/nhscoreprinciples.aspx):

- Principle 1 – comprehensive service available to all
- Principle 2 – access to the NHS is based on clinical need, not on the ability to pay
- NHS value: 'everyone counts'

All these could be said to reiterate critical theory's concerns with equity, empowerment and emancipation.

Reflection 2.12

You might like to consider how possible it is for you as a student nurse to be empowered. Would this situation change if you qualify as a staff nurse or would you be more empowered as a ward manager?

Going further, thinking about the wider context of the NHS and reflecting on your experiences as a student nurse to date, are all services based on clinical need and not the ability to pay? Is the service comprehensive?

In other words, how likely is it that empowerment and emancipation are meaningfully at the heart of the NHS?

We now need to consider what patients need to emancipate themselves from and what is it about the doctor–patient relationship that is oppressive. To do so we will explore the medical model and medicalisation.

The medical model and medicalisation

The term medical model is imprecise but useful nonetheless. It refers to a framework of assumptions that are thought to underpin the doctor–patient relationship, and that rely on the training doctors receive in how to diagnose and treat illness. Doctors use a set of procedures including: taking a history, physically examining the patient, requesting other tests if needed, diagnosis, treatment, and prognosis with and without treatment. However, and this is important, doctors are not trained to focus on health by and large; therefore they tend to be experts at medicine but not at healthcare necessarily. Doctors view the human body as an object, a machine that at times needs repair; the medical model understands the human body scientifically, as a physical body. And as the sociologist Irving Goffman suggested, in this relationship the doctor is the expert and the patient the object. Goffman referred to this service as 'medical servicing'. Of course, nowadays many doctors (quite rightly) would argue that they are trained more holistically than Laing and Goffman imply. Nevertheless, there is a certain truth to the idea that medicine is a science and that the physical body assumes precedence over the mental, emotional or psychological bodies. You may have been taught about the body and health using the 'bio-psycho-social' model, which is a response to the critique that the medical model is a too narrow and oppressive way to approach human health and illness.

Both Laing and Goffman were both interested in mental illness – Laing was a psychiatrist famous for criticising psychiatry and Goffman wrote an influential book called *Asylums* (1961) which detailed the institutionalising effect of mental institutions or hospitals. And it is in mental health nursing and learning disability nursing that one can see how restrictive an overly scientific, physical model of understanding illness might be.

The term medicalisation was first coined by Ivan Illich, who was not a critical theorist but his observations are a useful place to start. He was interested in how social institutions (structures) affected individuals. So he studied modern medicine and suggested that a characteristic of modern medicine was the way it had spread its activities to areas beyond doctors' original training (above), such as the processes of birth, which were traditionally under the control of midwives (and women), and death, which traditionally took place in the home and was private. The emerging influence of and then control by medicine over childbirth is commonly understood to be because obstetrics results in safer births. Yet while modern obstetric practice may have improved the safety of birth, better hygiene, diet and birth control are equally important; and along with medical involvement comes medical *control*. So as doctors increased their role in birth, so they increased their control over birth and women (Ehrenreich and English, 2005, 2010).

But that's not the only problem with medicalisation. Illich argued that medicalisation had resulted in iatrogenesis: doctor-generated illness or the harmful effects of medical treatments. These included:

- clinical iatrogenesis – unwanted side-effects of medications, medical malpractice, ignorance or neglect;
- social iatrogenesis – medicine sponsors sickness and reinforces a morbid society that encourages people to become consumers of curative, preventive, industrial and environmental medicine;
- cultural iatrogenesis – societies weaken because people's responses to suffering, impairment and death are weakened by medicine through over-medicalisation.

In other words medicine makes people sick.

So far, we have argued that as well as class and gender inequalities, and inequalities due to ethnicity, people's health may be affected by the power that is located with medicine as a framework for understanding illness (the medical model) and, as a consequence, power that is ascribed to medical practitioners (medicalisation). We can see how critical theorists build on Marxist and Weberian theories of social divisions due to class and their resulting inequalities to argue that such social relations are also based on knowledge which is itself biased in favour of those in power within societies. In other words, the bourgeoisie, who own the means of production, also influence the production of knowledge to both shape and understand society. To continue our example of psychiatric illness, critical theorists would argue that understanding mental illness as a biochemical imbalance whose treatment is a drug manufactured by the pharmaceutical industry which is owned by the bourgeoisie are not unrelated coincidental facts but linkages between knowledge, the social relations of production and class inequalities.

Reflection 2.13

You might like to consider whether, 40 years after Illich's *Medical Nemesis*, doctors are still expanding their control over areas of our lives that aren't 'medical'. Do women have more control over childbirth than in the 1960/1970s? Do patients have more control over their health and decisions in illness? How far does government either encourage patients to make decisions or facilitate medical control over health and illness?

One of the ways in which critics of medicine and the medical profession have suggested that control is exerted over patients is through medical technologies such as ultrasound in pregnancy. Such forms of technological surveillance may be understood as forms of social control. Now consider Reflection 2.14.

Reflection 2.14   Pregnancy ultrasound as social control

Read the article by M. Wagner in *Midwifery Today*: Ultrasound: more harm than good? www.midwiferytoday.com/articles/ultrasoundwagner.asp.

Ultrasound in pregnancy has been an accepted part of routine ante-natal care worldwide, yet it is also a good example of iatrogenesis because, in the eyes of many midwives and pregnant women, it medicalises what should be a 'natural' process.

In the light of our discussion here about the ways in which knowledge, power, the ownership of the means of production and class relations are produced and reproduced, pay particular attention to what Wagner says about:

- The medical model – viewing the human body as an object: 'The ultrasound story begins in July 1955 when an obstetrician in Scotland, Ian Donald, borrowed an industrial ultrasound machine used to detect flaws in metal and tried it out on some tumours, which he had removed previously, using a beefsteak as the control. He discovered that different tumours produced different echoes. Soon Donald was using ultrasound not only for abdominal tumours in women but also on pregnant women.'
- Medicalisation – spread of medical activities: '"ultrasound is now no longer a diagnostic test applied to a few pregnancies regarded on clinical grounds as being at risk. It can now be used to screen all pregnancies and should be regarded as an integral part of antenatal care" (Campbell & Little, 1980)'.
- Medical control – technology or intervention seen as standard practice: 'After a technology has spread widely in clinical practice, the next step is for health policymakers to accept it as standard care financed by the official health sector.'
- Knowledge – understanding how knowledge emerges to promote ways of behaving and in this case forgetting the 'distinction between its [ultrasound scan's] selective use for specific indications and its routine use as a screening procedure'.
- Links to means of production owned by the bourgeoisie (wealthy): 'In many countries, the commercial application of ultrasound scanning during pregnancy is widespread, offering "baby look" and "fun ultrasound" in order to "meet your baby" with photographs and home videos.'

Chapter summary

In Marxist theory, the patient is obliged to comply through the unequal class relations that shape the doctor–patient relationship. In a doctor–patient relationship where the doctor and patient are from the same class position, then the patient will be given preferential treatment (Willems et al., 2005).

To some extent health professionals have begun to respond to patient activism and it is now more common to talk about patient adherence rather than compliance, which retains a hint of the doctor knows best but some recognition that the doctor can't have it all his way.

However, critical theorists go further than adherence to talk about resistance. In critical theory, and for Illich too, while the doctor–patient relationship is unequal and, for Illich, iatrogenic, patients need not comply; they can resist. To that extent there is potential for emancipation and empowerment.

Going further

See Dillon (2010) (cited below) for a further explanation of Marx's ideas or Jessop's chapter in Stone (2008) *Key Sociological Thinkers*, 2nd edition. Basingstoke, Hants, UK: Palgrave Macmillan.

You might want to read the Preface to *A Contribution to the Critique of Political Economy* for yourselves: www.marxists.org/archive/marx/works/1859/critique-pol-economy/preface.htm.

If you want to know about global exploitation of workers, try looking at this website: www.theguardian.com/global-development/poverty-matters/2013/may/16/bangladesh-garment-workers-exploitation-slavery.

See Tudor Hart's original piece in the *Lancet*: www.thelancet.com/journals/lancet/article/PIIS0140-6736(71)92410-X/abstract.

Giddens, A. and Sutton, P.W. (2012) *Sociology*. Cambridge: Polity Press.

The Royal College of Nursing has produced the publication *Health Inequalities and the Social Determinants of Health*. It discusses social class, health inequalities and puts this in the context of the nurse's role in public health and current government policy which seeks to improve health inequalities: www.rcn.org.uk/about-us/policy-briefings/pol-0112.

Have a look at the Office of National Statistics website and see for yourself how health inequalities change over time, by social class, gender, age, ethnicity and area you live in: www.ons.gov.uk/ons/taxonomy/index.html?nscl=Population#tab-overview.

See Graham Scambler's blog www.grahamscambler.com/the-assault-on-our-nhs/ for ongoing comment on current debates around the NHS.

References

Arber, S.L. (2013) Gender, health and aging: continuity and change after 2 decades. British Sociological Association *Medical Sociology Online* 7(3): 28–37.

Bolton, S. and Wibberley, G. (2014) Domiciliary care: the formal and informal process. *Sociology* 48(4): 683–697.

Busfield, J. (2010) A pill for every ill: explaining the expansion of medicine use. *Social Science & Medicine* 70(6): 934–941. Available at: www.sciencedirect.com.ezproxy.mdx.ac.uk/science/article/pii/S0277953609008193

Campbell, S. and Little, D. (1980) Clinical potential of real-time ultrasound. In M. Bennett and S. Campbell (eds) *Real-time Ultrasound in Obstetrics*. Oxford: Blackwell Scientific Publications.

Carper, B. (1978) Fundamental patterns of knowing in nursing. *Advances in Nursing Science* 1(12): 13–24.

Dahlgren, G. and Whitehead, M. (1993) Tackling inequalities in health: what can we learn from what has been tried? Working paper prepared for the King's Fund International Seminar on Tackling Inequalities in Health, Ditchley Park, Oxfordshire, September, accessible in: Dahlgren, G. and Whitehead, M. (2007) European strategies for tackling social inequities in health: levelling up Part 2. Copenhagen: WHO Regional Office for Europe. Available at: www.euro.who.int/__data/assets/pdf_file/0018/103824/E89384.pdf.

Dillon, M. (2010) *Introduction to Sociological Theory: Theorists, Concepts and Their Applicability to the Twenty-First Century*. Chichester: Wiley-Blackwell.

Ehrenreich, B. and English, D. (2005) For her own good: two centuries of the experts' advice to women. New York: Feminist Press.

Ehrenreich, B. and English, D. (2010) *Witches, Midwives and Nurses*, 2nd edition. New York: Feminist Press.

Giddens, A. and Sutton, P. W. (2012) *Sociology*. Cambridge: Polity Press.

Goffman, E. (1961) *Asylums*. New York: Doubleday and Anchor.

Goodman, B. (2014) Paulo Freire and the pedagogy of the oppressed. *Nurse Education Today* 34, 1055–1056

Griffith, D. (1987) Nonmarket labor processes in an advanced capitalist economy. *American Anthropologist* 89(4): 838–852

Grundy, E. and Holt, G. (2005) Health inequalities in the older population. *Health Variations* 7. Available at: www.lancaster.ac.uk/fass/projects/hvp/pdf/nl7art2.pdf.

Illich, I. (1974) *Medical Nemesis*. London: Calder & Boyars.

Institute of Medicine (2001) *Crossing the Quality Chasm: A New Health System for the 21st Century*. Available at: https://iom.nationalacademies.org/~/media/Files/Report%20Files/2001/Crossing-the-Quality-Chasm/Quality%20Chasm%202001%20%20report%20brief.pdf (Retrieved 26 November 2012).

Jewson, N. (1976) The disappearance of the sick-man from medical cosmology, 1770–1870. *Sociology* 10(2): 225–247.

Marx, K. (1859) *A Contribution to the Critique of Political Economy*. Moscow: Progress Publishers.

Medical Research Council (1994) *Topic Review: the Health of the UK's Elderly People*. London: MRC.

National Life Tables (2011–13) www.ons.gov.uk/ons/rel/lifetables/national-life-tables/2011-2013/index.html.

Office for National Statistics (2011) *General Lifestyle Survey*. Available at: www.ons.gov.uk/ons/rel/ghs/general-lifestyle-survey/2011/index.html.

Office for National Statistics (2013) *Women in the Labour Market*. Available at: www.ons.gov.uk/ons/rel/lmac/women-in-the-labour-market/2013/rpt---women-in-the-labour-market.html.

Oldroyd, J., Bannerjee, M., Heald, A. and Cruickshank, K. (2005) Diabetes and ethnic minorities. *Post Graduate Medical Journal* 81: 486–490. Available at: http://pmj.bmj.com/content/81/958/486.full.

Porter, S. (1998) *Social Theory and Nursing Practice*. Basingstoke: Palgrave Macmillan.

Scambler, G. (2012) Resistance in unjust times: Archer, structured agency and the sociology of health inequalities. *Sociology* 47: 142–156.

Steptoe, A., Wardle, J., Lipsey, Z., Mills, R., Olier, G., Jarvis, M. and Kirschbaum, C. (1998) A longitudinal study of work load and variations in psychological well-being, cortisol, smoking, and alcohol consumption. *Annals of Behavioral Medicine* 20(2): 84–91.

Tiggle, D.J. (2007) Treating desires not diseases: a pill for every ill and an ill for every pill? *Drug Discovery Today* 12(3–4): 161–166. Available at: www.sciencedirect.com.ezproxy.mdx.ac.uk/science/article/pii/S1359644606004831

Tudor Hart, J. (1971) The inverse care law. *The Lancet* 297(7696): 405–412.

Willems, S., De Maesschalck, S., Deveugele, M., Derese, A. and De Maeseneer, J. (2005) Socio-economic status of the patient and doctor-patient communication: does it make a difference? *Patient Education and Counselling* 56: 139–146.

3

Becoming a nurse

Michael Traynor

Issue/concern

This chapter examines how everyday events contribute to professional socialisation.

Here's a list of a few things a student nurse might start off feeling nervous about but gradually come to accept as natural:

- finding your way to placement sites;
- wearing strange clothes;
- shift work;
- unfamiliar and sinister smells;
- needing to make relationships with more experienced and senior colleagues, some of whom seem to take a dislike to students;
- not knowing how to talk to patients;
- not knowing anything;
- wondering whether you have made the right choice;
- assignments;
- new vocabulary – some of it in ancient languages;
- books about sociology.

Chapter outline

This chapter introduces the idea of professional socialisation by:

- Presenting an example of key sociological work on the topic
- Reviewing the basic concept of socialisation in society and in the professions

- Discussing what is said to make professions distinct from other occupations, including professional regulation
- Finishing with an example of a micro-sociological examination of the effect of socialisation on a group of student nurses, 'listening more carefully'
- A consideration of the contribution of social media to professional identity in nursing.

Introduction: key sociological work on the topic

In 1961 *Boys in White* (Becker et al., 1961) appeared. The Soviet Union put the first man in space and the average price of a house in the UK was £2770.[1] Push-button zebra crossings started to appear for the first time. *Boys in White*, an account of research by American sociologist Howard Becker and his colleagues, described the rite of passage that US school graduates went through to become first medical students and then doctors, climbing, along the way, into clothes, lab coats and various other articles, all in the medical symbolic colour of white. And though there were a few women going into medicine, most of them were boys,[2] gradually learning how to be 'medical men'. In the sixties, perhaps the heyday of the professions, those wishing to enter them and to gain their lucrative benefits had to endure longer and longer training, and decide to aim for them at an increasingly young age. Becker and colleagues set out, by closely following a number of medical students in one university, to discover 'what medical school did to medical students'. Their research, unlike much research you will read today, had only 'unstructured techniques' but it had a commitment to a sociological principle, that the researchers were interested in questions of a collective kind, in what happened to medical students by virtue of the fact that they shared in a structured set of social activities. They investigated what the students themselves were concerned about and they focused on what caused them problems on the basis that when things go well, people tend to be unreflective. By studying these things they aimed to build an overall model of the medical school where they could single out recurring elements from the mass of concrete events they observed and asked about. *Boys in White* has become a classic, a reference point for many subsequent studies of how ordinary people gradually become members of professional groups, including nursing. This is socialisation.

This chapter sets out the first of our investigations of the taken for granted. The 'taken for granted' on this occasion takes the form of the processes that you and your colleagues are likely to be participating in as students and new nurses as you move during the three years of your programme from rabbit in the headlights to calm, confident practitioner.

---

[1]At the time of writing, the average house price in the UK is £250,000 and the starting annual salary of a nurse is a little over £21,000.

[2]At roughly the same time that *Boys in White* appeared, a study of the organisation of nursing work and how nurses are socialised into that organisation was carried out by Isolbel Menzies (1960). It did not go down well at the time, which is all the more reason to search it out.

Your experiences

Most students and new nurses speak about experiencing nervousness and apprehension at some point in their programme or career, mixed with the satisfaction of doing a job that can make a difference to people's lives and the stimulation that arises in work where no two days are the same (http://targetjobs.co.uk/career-sectors/healthcare/290063-life-as-a-student-nurse). Perhaps surprisingly, it is at least partly through the fear, disorientation, loss of a sense of former identity and even humiliations that socialisation does its work (Schein, 1988).

Even further back than *Boys in White*, and in what is perhaps the medieval equivalent of today's young professionals, novices who joined monasteries, nunneries and religious orders went through initiation rites such as shaving their heads, wearing strange clothes and taking up new names. These practices symbolised the loss of a previous life and the beginning of a fundamentally new identity. In some ways tough coursework and the extremes of anxiety experienced in early clinical settings, with little support from staff who seem to have grown indifferent to students' fears, have a similar effect. The fundamental unfamiliarity and terror make you highly susceptible to socialisation, wanting, to put it simply, to fit in and find approval. This kind of regime, whether achieved as a deliberate strategy (some old-fashioned clinicians think this is an unproblematic way to introduce novices to professional work), or more by accident and neglect, can also bring about extremely close bonds between novices. Often those bonds can give rise to peer-group norms that are based on critique of those in authority. While this norm of critique is understandable, necessary and probably appropriate, it can also eventually prove unhelpful for reasons we will suggest to you later.

Socialisation in more detail: socialisation in society

In order to fully understand the concept of professional socialisation, we first need to step a long way back from thinking about the professions. According to some researchers, humans, unlike most non-human animals, produce infants that need to understand the culture that they are born into for survival itself (Macionis and Gerber, 2011). A child learning how to use the language it hears around it to make its needs known is one simple example. Sociologists as well as psychologists and philosophers have developed theories about how the human individual only develops identity through membership of groups. George Herbert Mead (1863–1931), for example, claimed that the 'self' is not present at birth but is only developed in social interaction with others (Mead, 1913). Through copying and reward – and punishment – children learn how to behave in a family and in other social units, for example in their sexual behaviour, table manners and respect for authority (Fox, 2012). Because this kind of socialisation reflects and maintains a group's existing values and ways of understanding the world and acting in it, those from a range of cultures and backgrounds as well as boys and girls will tend to feel it natural to behave in different ways once they have grown up and become well-functioning members of those societies. Sociologists such as Harold Garfinkel and Harvey Sacks[3] both revealed the taken-for-granted rules of everyday behaviour and conversation that members of different groups take enormous, though usually unconscious, pains to obey and promote. Garfinkel and Sacks and those who have worked in their tradition show that individuals continually work on their self-presentation for the social order to hold in place. Some of this work has focused on health professionals and we will return that these studies later.

As hinted at just now, boys and girls are, in virtually every society, socialised to behave and experience the world in different ways and these depend largely on the values and practices already existing in those societies. The debate still continues but we would like to suggest that many of the qualities believed by many to be innate or biologically caused in either gender can be seen to be the result of cultural belief and practice. As preparation for thinking about socialisation in nursing and health-care it is important to be aware of gender socialisation for the simple reason that the vast majority of nurses happen to be women. It is likely that the way the profession is understood and understands itself is going to in some way reflect, or perhaps work against, the way women are viewed by society at large. One unavoidable fact about gender socialisation is that, if socialisation tends to support the existing values of society, then in societies where one group has been able to dominate and hold power over others, those others will tend to get a rough time from socialisation. And many believe most human societies to be patriarchal. The Oxford Dictionary has a useful definition of patriarchy:

> A system of society or government in which men hold the power and women are largely excluded from it. (www.oxforddictionaries.com/definition/english/patriarchy)

Many global organisations have drawn attention to the disadvantage still faced by women worldwide as a result of patriarchy. For example, women do two-thirds of the world's work but earn only 10 per cent of the world's income and own 1 per cent of the world's property (UNICEF, 2007). In addition, they are far more likely than men to be on the receiving end of a spectrum of sexual violence from dismissive or patronising attitudes to murder and rape (World Health Organization and London School of Hygeine and Tropical Medicine, 2013). Gender socialisation is also reflected in the world of work, where women are over-represented in certain types of work – those generally with low economic value and status – and under-represented in others. This can in turn affect the career

---

[3]Harold Garfinkel (1917–2011) worked, for the most part, at the University of California, Los Angeles. He was the founder of 'ethnomethodology', the detailed study of how members of particular groups (it could be jurors or surfers or even people standing in a queue) adopt particular methods to make sense of and make sense in the societies or contexts they find themselves in. Harvey Sacks (1935–1975) was influenced by ethnomethodology and developed a detailed – extremely detailed – approach to studying conversational interaction. His aim was similar to Garfinkel's, to discover the underlying rules that members of societies pay attention to when going about their everyday activities.

and educational expectations of women. We will return to women in 'caring' work when we discuss the professions later in this chapter.

Once we are aware of socialisation then we can see its effects everywhere. If gender socialisation might have an effect on occupational aspirations, then so might social class.

Reflection 3.1

We introduced the concept of social class in Chapter 2.

We suggest you use this 'class calculator' to find out which class you belong to at www.bbc.co.uk/news/magazine-22000973.

In the 1980s a survey found that children in families where the father was in a professional or managerial occupation were twice as likely to aspire to a similar occupation than children with working-class fathers (Furlong, 1993). More recent studies suggest that the link between British children's social class and their educational attainment is well established (Goldthorpe 2003; DES, 2005) and that there is little evidence that the class-based attainment gap is closing at primary level (DES, 2005). At secondary level the difference in achievement in terms of class remains the widest of all the forms of social stratification (Baars and ISC (University of Manchester), 2010: 2).

No discussion of socialisation is complete without a mention of multiculturalism. It is important to discuss this concept because health-service work involves working alongside and treating people from a diverse range of cultural backgrounds. Multiculturalism is a common, and for some controversial, term often referred to in Western liberal democracies. We can understand multiculturalism either as a simple description of the fact of cultural diversity within a particular society or as a set of policies that set out to enable and promote this diversity and work against the prejudice and disadvantage that might face those in minority groups in society.[4] In terms of individuals, one could say that those who have grown up in a white British non-religious working-class family may have been socialised in a different way from two neighbours one of whom is from a Muslim family originally from Pakistan and the other the child of African-Caribbean Evangelical Christians. Many aspects of their socialisation will be similar but some will be different. And multicultural policies set out to preserve that difference. However, there is also the assumption that members of every culture will find the values underpinning liberal democracies attractive. Multiculturalism encourages people to 'value diversity' but this can

---

[4]For a brief but useful investigation of whether UK multicultural policies have failed see Manning (2011).

sometimes mask an expectation that everyone must conform to liberal tolerant values, in public at least. For example, liberal values promote a welcoming of diversity in sexuality and sexual orientation but if you believe that your religion teaches that homosexuality is a sin, a look at recent news stories will show you that it is possible that you will lose your job in the UK public sector if you tell a gay colleague about your beliefs (*Guardian*, 2014).[5]

Professional socialisation

Having introduced the concept of socialisation in society as a whole we can now think about the processes specific to professional socialisation.

Reflection 3.2

See what the RCN says about socialisation here: http://www2.rcn.org.uk/ development/practice/professional_attitudes_and_behaviours/socialisation

You can see that even your choice to consider nursing as a career has at least something to do with your socialisation. There is more to that choice than the account you possibly gave about personal experiences and personal attributes when you were interviewed. Perhaps more interesting though, is to consider how far the worldview and values you have developed in your socialisation to date (in your family or social group, for example) are similar or different to the worldview and values at work in socialisation into nursing, the theory being that the more difference and dissonance between them, the tougher your experience might be. One obvious aspect of this is that you may have held some inaccurate beliefs about nursing work gained from the media before coming up against the reality. But there will be other more subtle disorientations at work such as expectations about acceptable and unacceptable uses of humour.

Returning to *Boys in White*, the authors use the term 'perspective' as part of their investigation of the culture of medical students. The way they open up this term helps us to understand professional socialisation. By perspective they mean the 'co-ordinated set of ideas and actions a person uses in dealing with some problematic situation … a person's ordinary way of thinking and feeling about and acting in such a situation' (p. 34). So what is a problematic situation? A 'long-range'

---

[5]See www.christianconcern.com/media/rod-liddle-interviews-sarah-mbuyi for an interview with a nursery nurse who was dismissed after expressing this view, as well as an insightful intervention by Peter Tatchell, political campaigner and champion of LGBT rights.

perspective is what has brought an individual into a particular situation. This might be the perspective that medical school is a good thing (or that medicine is a good thing) and that it is necessary to finish medical school in order to practise medicine. Given this, a student enters medical school and, in terms of the long-range perspective of the necessity to successfully complete the course, is faced with a number of problems which demand short-term perspectives. Becker and colleagues go on to say that group perspectives develop when people find themselves 'in the same boat' regarding these problems. Let's translate one of their examples into nursing education. If you had carried out their study among nursing students in any particular university you might have noticed that students are in agreement that they need to put all their efforts into staying on the right side of lecturers and qualified staff, including mentors. Because, according to the shared belief, these groups can be unpredictable in what they want of you and can be out to find fault with you, and students can lie and 'cheat' in order to please lecturers, qualified staff and mentors.[6] And they want to please them because of the necessity of passing the course and it is necessary to pass the course in order to qualify and practise as a nurse. So, while 'official' nursing socialisation may be concerned with producing nurses who 'respect patients' dignity' and are 'caring', there are other aspects of socialisation at work that are little discussed but experienced as more urgent by student nurses.[7]

As we have already mentioned, professional socialisation involves both explicit teaching and informal, more-or-less unconscious, learning (some writers talk about 'internalising values and beliefs' (Davis, 1975)). Both of these are at work in the university and in clinical settings. Professions themselves are usually keen to identify the positive and relatively formal aspects of socialisation and to condemn obviously unacceptable parts but are silent about some of the more ambiguous informal aspects. The following table lists some of the features of professional socialisation in nursing. We have given some examples and put them into categories. In the fourth column we have placed activities and attitudes that reflect uncomfortable realities of nursing work. They are perhaps the hardest to talk about publicly because they contain within them a seed of something destructive to the profession's image but they represent necessary practice to get the work done. Being socialised in nursing, and medicine, involves learning how to act in this column.[8]

---

[6]Becker's illustrative example is of the student who fails to do laboratory work on a patient's blood but who copies other results and draws some blood from the patient too in case the senior doctor checked up on him (p. 38).

[7]An example from nursing: in focus groups with student nurses conducted by one of us, a great many students were frank about turning a blind eye to what they considered poor practice they had witnessed in order not to alienate ward nurses whom they would rely on for good reports and to successfully pass placements.

[8]For more about this see Chambliss (1996).

Reflection 3.3

Consider the categories in which we have placed some nursing activities, skills or knowledge. What do you particularly think about those in the right-hand column?

	Positive	Negative	Ambiguous
Skills	Patient care skills such as recording vital signs	Incompetent in patient care skills	Skill in asking to borrow needed equipment
Knowledge	Anatomy and physiology	Inadequate knowledge	Which other members of nursing or medical staff to avoid working with
Behaviour	How to present a neat competent professional appearance	Speaking disrespectfully to patients	How to talk about patients 'backstage' to other nurses
Internalising values and beliefs	Individualised care: 'the patient is at the centre of all we do'	Routinised or institutionalised care	Responsibility to maintain patient throughput and prioritise requests for attention
	To empathise with patient distress	Lack of empathy leading to neglect	To establish distance from strong emotion and routinise daily dramatic events in order to work effectively

What are professions anyway and why do people want to join them?

If becoming a member of a new profession is so difficult, for the reasons discussed above, then it is clear that socialisation depends on you having a strong motivation to join the group otherwise you would walk away, as some do during training. In fact dropping out, 'attrition', is surprisingly common and a problem that those who commission and pay for nursing education, and the universities that provide it, are extremely keen to tackle (Lintern, 2013). Exactly what a profession is and the rewards that its members are given has been discussed by sociologists for at least one hundred years. Which occupations can be considered to have gained this enviable status is also the subject of much debate – as well as how they did it. Medicine has been considered as the exemplar profession while nursing has usually been described as an aspiring or a semi-profession.

The earliest sociological theories about the professions that were developed during the early years of the twentieth century saw them in terms of their positive contribution to the societies in which they developed and often tried to define what differentiated a profession from all the other occupations. The professions were sources of expertise (for example legal or medical) available to society and the professionals within them possessed not only a unique body of knowledge (obtained through often lengthy training) but an ethic of service to their clients and an altruism that protected lay people from the potential self-interest of the professions. These types of understanding have been labelled structural functionalist and are associated with writers such as Talcott Parsons (see our discussion of 'the sick role' in Chapter 2). He contrasted professional 'disinterestedness' with a prevalent concern for self-interest (though clearly in the 1950s when he was writing there was little conception of women professionals): 'The professional man is not thought of as engaged in the pursuit of his personal profit, but in performing services to his patients or clients, or to impersonal values like the advancement of science' (Parsons, 1954: 35).

From approximately the 1970s onwards writers began to move on from rather static discussions of professional traits to explore a more dynamic and perhaps less positive side of professionalism. Writers such as Magali Larson, for example in *The Rise of Professionalism* (1977), focused on the professionalisation project that members of emerging professions engage in, in order to clear a space for themselves in a market for their services.[9] As previously mentioned, mid-nineteenth-century British medicine has been seen as an exemplar of a successfully established profession. When this 'project' is successful, the result is a legally enforceable monopoly often accompanied by significant social status and financial reward for professionals. For example, if you were to start doing the work of a doctor – or nurse – without the legitimate training, you could end up in prison. No wonder the Boys in White were prepared to cheat on their tutors, endure their wrath and work long hours in order to become doctors. But today the so-called professional traits – the unique body of theoretical knowledge, autonomy in work, control of entry to the profession – are more likely to be discussed in terms of their symbolic value that less established professional groups aspire to and work hard to achieve (Collins, 1979). Many writers of nursing's early history use this approach to explain how the profession's leaders in the nineteenth and early twentieth centuries in Britain explicitly copied medicine's tactics in order to gain professional standing. For example, characters such as Ethel Bedford-Fenwick (1857–1947) campaigned for a nationally recognised training for nurses leading to state registration. (She had the honour of being the first nurse on the register after the Nurses Registration Act was passed in 1919.)

Nursing's 'professional project' involved an attempt by Bedford-Fenwick and others to establish a monopoly over the provision of 'nursing' skills and competencies to achieve 'occupational closure'. The reward of their 30-year campaign for registration was control over the supply of nurses. This was achieved by including on the register only those individuals who had gone through a uniform system of

---

[9]Other writers explored the negative effects of medicine in terms of 'medicalisation' of an increasing number of life events (such as birth and death). See Illich (1977) or Kennedy (1981). See also Chapter 2 in this book.

education and excluding all the others who practised in work that many at that time would have considered nursing. In other words, this project involved a credentialist claim for nursing work; that is, you need the credential of registration to be allowed to work as a nurse. Some have argued that registration enabled the socio-economically privileged leaders of nursing (for example Mrs Bedford-Fenwick – see Chapter 5 for more detail – was the daughter of a wealthy doctor and the member of a well-connected family) the opportunity to reshape the profession along class lines. Registration, they anticipated, would also enable 'self-government' as opposed to the 'subjugation' of nurses by medical men. Sociologist Anne Witz presents such a project as evidence that women can mount effective challenges to patriarchal systems, challenges that have the potential to liberate women from the label of 'semi-professionals'. However, nurses were not entirely successful. Witz noted that many unqualified workers continued to do work that could be defined as nursing work and that nurses themselves engaged in duties that could be considered as supporting or auxiliary work (Witz, 1992).

The label 'semi-professions' was applied by Amitai Etzioni and colleagues writing in 1969 to three occupations: teaching, social work and nursing. The chapter on nursing was written by Fred Katz who believed that hospital nursing and medicine were caught in a rigid caste system of medical superiority. He concluded that the nurse 'has no clearly formulated body of professional knowledge that is recognized and accepted by others' (Etzioni, 1969: 62). This work, of course, is old and Katz's studies were already dated and to the contemporary reader seem full of assumption and social prejudice. Nevertheless, his chapter, and the book as a whole, touches on something that has not gone away, namely that occupations made up largely of women struggle for recognition and reward.

Most studies of nursing, medicine and professionalism emphasise the role of gender in this relationship. One contribution to this topic is the suggestion that the idea of medical professional autonomy relies on a blindness to the work of, usually female, clerical, nursing or other health-service staff whose work enables doctors to do their job and to have the brief encounter with the individual patient, at the heart of this concept of professionalism, for which the patient may wait many hours or even months or years. Some sociologists have argued that the whole notion of being a professional and working in an organisation is 'gendered' male because its bureaucratic features require a kind of impartial, formalised, disembodied, rational approach that many have seen as reflecting stereotypical male values. Faced with this, writers including Celia Davies[10] have argued that nursing needs a radically different concept of what it is to be a profession (Davies, 1995).

If in its early years nursing explicitly copied medicine's professionalising tactics, by the middle of the twentieth century many in the profession were doing everything they could to differentiate the profession from medicine. The issue was that doctors had been heavily involved in the selection and training of nurses, sending uncomfortable messages about its subjugation. In the unchallenged patriarchal days

---

[10]Davies is a feminist sociologist with a long involvement in studying medicine and nursing. She was one of the architects of a radical overhaul of nurse education in the late 1990s and has written about gender and nursing's 'professional predicament'.

of the 1940s this might have felt natural but 30 years later, with the emergence of feminism in the meantime, such reliance on medical men was feeling increasingly anachronistic, unacceptable and unnecessary. Many academic nurses were calling for nursing practice and education to be based on a specifically *nursing* knowledge base which was neither watered-down medicine nor a patchwork of borrowed theories. This effort gave rise to many responses. Some took the form of rather crude attempts to appropriate medical symbols such as the development of 'nursing diagnoses' (diagnosis, along with prescribing medicines being key features of medical practice), involving the compiling of a vast international system of classification to be used by nurses.

Reflection 3.4   Nursing diagnoses – useful or just bizarre?

Most descriptions of nursing diagnoses take pains to emphasise their distinctness from medical diagnoses and their holistic and 'patient-centred' character as opposed to medical diagnoses which are described as disease focused. For example, see http://allnurses.com/nursing-student-assistance/student-resources-nursing-424826.html.

One nursing diagnosis is disturbed energy field: 'Disruption of the flow of energy surrounding a person's being that results in disharmony of the body, mind and/or spirit' (NANDA International, 2014).

On your next clinical placement, why not try informing the ward sister that you suspect one of your patients is suffering from disturbed energy field?

Others were more radical though more risky, with an attempt to identify a specifically nursing epistemology (Schultz and Meleis, 1988); that is, an attempt to recognise the unique features of how nurses come to know what they know that differentiates them from other groups. We leave it to you to judge how useful and interesting such projects might be for learning and practice. The point is that these can be understood as part of an overall professionalising strategy, with some rooted in the particular times and cultures where they were devised.

Professional regulation

Now that we have discussed cultural and professional socialisation and introduced some sociological views of the professions, we need to return to professional regulation and talk in more depth about it as this too operates within a social context. To work in the UK as a nurse, midwife or specialist community public health nurse you need to register with the Nursing and Midwifery Council (NMC) and, at the time of writing, renew your registration every year. The NMC will have shaped the course you are taking (or have taken) and set out what you have to do to stay practising as a nurse; it has formulated a code of conduct and can discipline you if you either perform poorly as a nurse (to the extent that it can be argued that you have broken the code) or threaten to bring the profession into disrepute by being convicted of criminal acts unconnected to your nursing work. As we mentioned earlier, state-sponsored professional self-regulation is perhaps the ultimate prize for any aspiring profession; however, how far this is 'self'-regulation and how far the regulator is simply an agent of government discipline has shifted over the last 50 years. The NMC, for example, states that it is independent from government (Nursing and Midwifery Council, 2013) but it is clearly under strong pressure from successive governments who appoint its members and, recently, its chair. From perhaps the 1960s onwards the respect and power allowed to traditional professions alongside other authority figures (vicars, bank managers and white middle-class men in general) was being challenged. Professional regulators like other conservative institutions were able to resist this change for many years. For example in 1979 27 out of 33 members of the UKCC, the successor to the General Nursing Council, were nurses. Of the remaining six, two were doctors and four 'lay' members with financial or educational expertise to offer. The Council was seen as on the side of the professionals; however, during the 1980s Margaret Thatcher's government commissioned management consultants JM Consulting to look at possible changes to the way that the allied health professions (AHPs are usually considered to include physiotherapy, occupational therapy and ten other professional groups) were regulated. The review did not include medical regulation. However, in 1997 New Labour used the same consultants to carry out a review of the regulation of nursing and midwifery (JM Consulting Ltd, 1998). The report considered that nursing and midwifery regulation was too inward looking and that its workings did not adequately involve lay people. It considered this degree of insularity as outmoded in a society where it was no longer realistic to consider the public as having too little understanding of the work of professionals to participate in their regulation on a par with them. The report's repeated claim was that the key duty of professional regulators is to protect the public. The present regulator, the NMC, took over from its predecessor organisation in 2002 with stronger lay representation and warnings not to be 'overly sympathetic' to professionals.

These changes were made more palatable and perhaps given a sense of urgency by a number of medical scandals that emerged during the 1990s. One was the 'Bristol Inquiry'. The Bristol Royal Infirmary and the Bristol Royal Hospital for Sick Children were teaching hospitals linked with Bristol University's Medical School and looked after patients with heart disease. From the late 1980s concerns were expressed about the mortality rate for particular surgical procedures for babies with congenital heart disease. The concerns turned into complaints to the General Medical Council (GMC) and two surgeons were struck off and another was disciplined. A public inquiry was opened in 1998 (Kennedy and Bristol Royal Infirmary, 2000). A second scandal concerned the murders by GP Harold Shipman of up to 200 of his patients, mostly elderly women (Chief Medical Officer, 2001). So, increased state involvement in professional regulation occurred during a period when it was likely to be harder to resist by the professions as these scandals were widely seen as inadequately dealt with by the medical regulator. It could be said that over a period of 150 years, the medical profession has changed from resembling a social elite with little accountability to starting to become a more scrutinised profession.

Since the early 2000s, however, the NMC has experienced a series of troubles. It has been the subject of a number of highly critical government reviews identifying poor record keeping, slow processes, poor training of its committee members and a culture of bullying. Partly as a result of these critiques, the NMC has had five heads in six years, not a good basis for stability and leadership. The current chair appointed by the government in 2012 is not a nurse but a senior civil servant with a history of rescuing failing organisations. Nevertheless, the NMC continues its work of managing the register and conducting fitness to practise panels. In 2012–2013 it received a little over 4,000 new referrals, and the largest proportion, about 40 per cent of these, come from the employers of nurses or midwives. Some have looked to statistics like this, along with the events described above, as evidence that within nursing professional self-regulation is increasingly looking like regulation by the state and its managerial agents (Cooke, 2012). We will be discussing the sometimes fraught relationship between the state and major professions along with managerialism in Chapter 8.

Looking closer at nurses: listening more carefully

So far we have been looking largely at the big picture: discussing the changing way that sociologists have defined and conceptualised the professions, including discussion of professional traits, the gaining and operation of professional power, professional regulation and the place of the professions in the 'social order'. Now we return to where we started, to socialisation, but change perspective and move in much closer to look at a study of how individual groups of professionals – nurses in this case – behave and enact, or perform, to use the words of some writers, being professionals. In contrast to Talcott Parsons, whose broadly framed ideas about professions we discussed earlier, other sociologists believed that terms, or rather assumptions, such as 'social order' in Parsons' work could obscure the actual local processes that established and maintained this social order. Harold Garfinkel and others working in his tradition were astonished by and sought to reveal the almost entirely taken-for-granted common-sense methods and procedures that members of various groups use to achieve order within their particular social context. Much of this work has focused on examinations of the details of everyday talk (by means of audio or video recordings) and, in particular, conversation on the basis that social life is realised through language and spoken interaction. The field is known as ethnomethodology, meaning, approximately, the study of members' methods (of making sense and maintaining order), and the detailed study of conversation is known, unsurprisingly, as conversation analysis (or CA). The two together are sometimes referred to as EMCA. A major project within CA work is the study of institutional talk and prominent among that is work looking at interaction between healthcare professionals and their patients and clients. Within this, in turn, analysts focus on the interactional accomplishment of institutional identities. For example, the use of the pronoun 'we' (by a single person – a doctor for instance) has been understood as an appeal to institutional rather than personal identity (Heritage, 1997) and so a claim to authority and distance. It is probably fair to say that EMCA researchers' interests lie on a continuum from a desire to understand more about how interaction in talk is accomplished at one end to a more applied focus on the other. This application can be described as using the tools and concepts of EMCA in an attempt to understand what is happening in institutions or how professional identity is accomplished from day to day in, for example, the clinic or at the bedside in actual interactions. Because analysts wish to study the minutiae of interaction they have developed an arcane (to those who don't know it) system of transcription of recorded talk. The system particularly enables interaction, that is turn-taking and its disruptions, pauses, changes in volume and pace, to be represented. See the excerpt below.

Researchers have used EMCA to examine the professional identity of nurses by looking at how they interact with their patients but also to see how they interact with each other. The following passage is taken from focus group research that one of us held with second-year student nurses, from mixed branches, at a mystery university. It is part of an ongoing research project that we will refer to throughout this book. The research aims to document students' motivations, expectations and experiences throughout their education in order to understand something about developing professional identity. To date we have held 14 groups with student nurses, midwives and healthcare support workers training to be assistant practitioners involving a total of 128 students. This passage is taken from a group that expressed a great deal of dissatisfaction about their placement experiences in hospital settings. Group members spoke about witnessing what they felt was poor patient care and cliquey and bullying behaviour from staff. They also expressed a strong conviction that they were very different from many staff that they had encountered and that they would use what they said were their higher standards, once qualified, to challenge poor practice. I asked whether they had any strategies for doing this effectively. The passage below shows one group member, Participant 4, responding to this question and starting to explain how she would behave if she found herself working in a setting where she witnessed poor standards of patient care. She says that after having established trust with her colleagues she would take a gradual approach to challenging these standards. Just to point out to the reader unfamiliar with this type of research, the focus is not so much on what the group members say, and whether we think it is sensible, truthful and so on, but on what we can learn from the interaction itself.[11] Spend a few minutes reading this excerpt of the transcript.

---

[11]The transcription of this section of the focus-group recording was kindly performed by Johanna Rendle-Short from Australian National University in Canberra.

1.	P4	but I think if I entered in a place like that,
2.		I would probably be: (0.4) try to (0.4) get
3.		>good rela::tionships< with- with the team
4.		that I work with,
5.		and then from then,
6.		I would just be (0.4) challenging, or (0.2) moving,
7.		or changing things (0.2) slowly, slowly,
8.		'cos you can't just (0.2) be (0.2)
9.		go to the ward and say, (0.2) yeah alright.
10.		I don't agree with this.
11.	P?	=mm=
12.	P4	=.h and then a people would start (0.2) like=
13.	P?	=((multiple [voices))=
14.	P9	[h- ho:w do you cope though.
15.		you go to a ward.
16.		you'll then see: (0.2) something you're not happy with.
17.		even if it's just a comment to a patient,
18.		or another member of staff.
19.		and you repo:rt it.=
20.		=or you pull them up on it,=
21.	P?	=yes.=
22.	P9	=and then, you're deemed the outsider,
23.		you're deemed the stirrer.
24.		and you're then the outsider. (0.2) of the group,=
25.	P?	=yeah.=
26.	P9	=of the shift. every shift.=
27.	P?	=mm=
28.	P9	=you're excluded.
29.		how do you deal with that.
30.		as a hu:man being. ((other voices in the background))
31.		not just as nu::rse,
32.		as a human being.
33.		>thinking back to when you were in school.<
34.		if you weren't in the in-crowd.
35.		and >you know,< even out with your friends,
36.		you know, if you're not always the lively one,
37.	P?	yeah.
38.	P9	ho:w do: you deal with that?
39.	P4	well (0.2) I- I guess it's quite ha:rd.
40.		it's quite hard [to deal with that.]
41.	P9	[I think it's] impossible.

As you can see, this method of transcription allows us to be aware of a number of interactional features that shed light on how this group functions. I will only mention a few of the features here. First, the numbers in brackets indicate pauses, measured in seconds, and P4's turns include many hesitations. During her first turn an unidentified speaker makes an overlapping utterance (indicated by = signs) but P4 is finally interrupted by a number of others (line 13) speaking simultaneously. P9's interruption emerges from these voices with an elongated 'ho:w' which establishes the start of her turn. Her interruption lasts until line 38. P4 then attempts to respond but her response is ended with P9's overlapping 'I think it's impossible'. During P9's interruption, other group members express agreement at lines 21, 25, 27 and 37. In other words, her challenge receives widespread support. P4's view is effectively silenced by P9 with the support of many group members.[12]

Stepping aside from the CA approach now, we might observe that P4 was attempting to make a constructive suggestion about how poor practice might be challenged; however, the dominant voices in the focus group ensure that a negativity about this prevails. We might even observe that the strong distinction between the 'in-crowd' and 'out-crowd' that P9 apparently deplores is actually enacted within this group and is used to silence a potentially constructive line of talk. What might this very brief look at CA and at a single example of data tell us about becoming a nurse? Before answering we need to remember the warnings about generalisation in research, and in qualitative research in particular, that are to be found in any research methods textbook. We would be foolish to draw conclusions about the whole profession from ten people who study together at a single university. However, if we were to find that this type of interaction was not atypical across the whole dataset of the other groups conducted as part of this research, and perhaps in evidence in other similar research, then we might begin to feel more confident to express some tentative conclusions. What about this: aspects of how nurses behave (or we could say elements of nursing culture) can be transmitted unwittingly from established nurses to newcomers to the profession. And part of that culture includes a preference for negativity rather than for solving problems, along with a focus on interpersonal conflict and subjective experience. Simplistic and partial as this conclusion may be, I do not think we can ignore it as part of socialisation. There is a lot more to say about professional socialisation in nursing, but the finding, if you agree that it is a finding, that members of a group participate in a behaviour that they are ostensibly distancing themselves from is a surprising one, worthy of note.

Societies have changed hugely since the first studies of professional socialisation. We now drag this chapter into the twenty-first century by discussing the nurse and social media.

---

[12]Other transcription used in this passage: 'greater than' and 'lesser than' signs enclose speeded-up talk; square brackets mark the start and end of overlapping speech aligned to mark the precise position of overlap; underlining indicates emphasis; the extent of underlining within individual words locates emphasis and also indicates how heavy it is.

Social media creates new networks

We end this chapter by discussing how far the rise of the Internet and social media have changed the process of becoming, and being, a nurse. We will not be discussing the effect on healthcare delivery of various health technologies, self-monitoring phone apps or aspects of telemedicine, but rather will focus on the impacts on professional identity. Many sociologists and commentators have written about the huge benefits and the associated risks of the rapid development of a radically connected society that these phenomena have given rise to (van Dijck, 2013). In many ways the risks are results of reliance on technology, such as when banking systems fail, but there are other more subtle types of 'digital risk', many to do with their impact on privacy and the rise in possibilities for surveillance (Beck, 2013). The mid-2000s saw the invention of the term 'Web 2.0' to indicate a change from 'one to many' (e.g. a website providing information) to 'many to many' communications on the Internet. The rise of platforms such as Facebook, Twitter and YouTube,[13] coupled with mobile technology that enables connection to the Internet from almost any location, has made it possible for individuals to continually post data online. Those who have been critical of the rise of a 'surveillance society' have pointed out how users of these technologies wittingly or unwittingly make intimate aspects of their lives available for recording and scrutiny by corporations who wish to target us for their products and services, by governments who wish to monitor their population's activities for reasons of national security, political advantage or paranoia, and by employers and potential employers who wish to examine the profile of employees or job candidates. The concerns of nursing organisations and National Health Service (NHS) employers tend to focus on the reputational risks associated with individuals who identify themselves as nurses posting content that they feel brings either the profession or particular organisations into disrepute.

Reflection 3.5

The RCN issued 'legal advice' for members using the Internet in 2009: http://www2.rcn.org.uk/newsevents/press_releases/uk/rcn_issues_new_guidance_on_internet_usage; and the NMC have guidance on the use of social media by nurses on their website at www.nmc-uk.org/Nurses-and-midwives/Regulation-in-practice/Regulation-in-Practice-Topics/Social-networking-sites/.

What do you think about this guidance? What do you think about the balance of personal freedom – including the ability to 'whistleblow', professional responsibility and reputational issues?

---

[13]There are other more professionally or academically orientated equivalents such as LinkedIn (https://uk.linkedin.com) and ResearchGate (www.researchgate.net).

However, one person's reputational risk can be another person's exposure of corruption. The 'Arab Spring', a wave of revolutionary demonstrations across the Arab world between 2010 and 2012, was said to be facilitated by the extensive use of social media. Social media and Internet-enabled mobile phones allowed revolutionaries not only to rapidly spread information and to organise but to transmit propaganda images in the form of amateur video shot on phones across the world to mobilise sympathies for their causes (Lindsey, 2013). The regimes under threat in some of these countries attempted to block access to these media (see www.westminster.ac.uk/__data/assets/pdf_file/0004/220675/WPCC-vol9-issue2.pdf), giving an idea of their power.

So while, in the UK, the use of social media by some nurses to intimidate or bully colleagues, or make disparaging remarks about patients, or boast about being drunk at work leads to well-publicised disciplinary actions, there are many intelligent Internet interventions by nurses that offer commentary on NHS policy and activity or use these networking opportunities to build positively focused virtual communities that can link like-minded individuals across diverse geographical areas.

It is risky to recommend any website or discussion group in particular as the Internet changes so quickly, but, at the time of writing, these are some interesting examples of social media developed by nurses to do what social media does best, which is to create a space for debate and the movement of information. At the moment, my favourite nursing blog is the grumbling appendix (https://grumbling appendix.wordpress.com/about/). It focuses on nursing in the British NHS, is authored by a practising nurse and describes itself as offering challenging, thought-provoking journalism. When most public figures in nursing and the NHS are going to great lengths to present a bad situation in a positive light, the grumbling appendix offers blistering critique with satirical humour. With less satire and more information giving, the student nurse blogging collective is the creation of two students (http://florencenursingtales.blogspot.co.uk/) and aims to promote the use of blogging and other social media by others (http://britainsnurses.co.uk/news/blog/the-bulletin/stnbc-welcome-to-the-student-nurse-blogger-collective). We Nurses (https://twitter.com/wenurses) uses Twitter for making connections between nurses, hosting Twitter chats and promoting the use of Twitter and other social media among nurses.[14] It runs regular chats on clinical or professional topics that can be joined from any location in real time, though the archives of the chat remain after the chat is over. Alongside blogs and other social media creations that are the work of real people, many corporations and institutions have launched their own, usually with the underlying aim of promoting their qualities and attracting market share. Many blogs with 'nurse' in the title turn out to be of this kind, whether they are published by universities or recruitment agencies or sponsored by publishers.

---

[14]Murthy (2010: 1061) offers the following definition of Twitter: '(1) users have a public profile in which they broadcast short public messages or updates whether they are directed to specific user(s) or not, (2) messages become publicly aggregated together across users, and (3) users can decide whose messages they wish to receive, but not necessarily who can receive their messages; this is in distinction to most social networks where following each other is bi-directional (i.e. mutual)'.

They can be a source of information but they are unlikely to have the vibrancy, humour, criticality or honesty of the best individual's work.

To return to socialisation and to end this chapter, we ask how the rise of social media might affect the process of becoming a nurse. First, it enables networks or conversations to develop irrespective of place and, often, time. Because of this the concept of community, and the possibility for support and solidarity, becomes expanded. Being a student nurse is not a position invested with a great deal of power, but today no student need be alone and unconnected. Second, though the benefits are exaggerated, social media offers some democratising opportunities. Although those with power, whether governments or large corporations, take up significant space on the Internet as well as influence with conventional media, many critical voices are now able to gain audiences in ways that were almost impossible in earlier times. Critiques and alternative views can be expressed but also evidence of corruption or corporate dishonesty, for example, can be instantly presented to a global audience. Third, because social media blurs the public/private divide, the 'backstage' stories (Goffman, 1959) that were previously shared in private between professionals may now be easily eavesdropped by the public and cause a great deal of offence, real and manufactured. Even government ministers resign after making this gaffe. We become professionals in this new place of visibility.

Chapter summary

In this chapter we have discovered that there is something surprising and perhaps counterintuitive about professional socialisation. Perhaps most notable is that professionals need, to an extent that would surprise and even shock the outsider, to routinise the dramatic. They do this in order to be able to do the work. Professional work is highly prized and aspiring entrants will act in unexpected ways in order not to jeopardise their entry. Student nurses have little power in NHS and nursing hierarchies; however, the appearance of social media can provide a forum for connection and support that can link those who might otherwise be isolated.

Going further

You can read about the NMC's work and remit on its website (www.nmc-uk.org) and see recent statistics on its fitness to practise work in Nursing and Midwifery Council (2013) *Nursing and Midwifery Council Annual Fitness to Practise Report 2012–2013*. London: The Stationery Office.

A comprehensive and accessible summary of CA processes can be found at the website of one of its leading European proponents, Paul ten Have, at www.paultenhave.nl/mica.htm.

Researchers at Loughborough University have summarised the transcription conventions used in this chapter at http://homepages.lboro.ac.uk/~ssca1/notation.htm.

For an example of the use of CA to examine the interactions between health professionals and their clients see the work of David Silverman (1997).

For a collection of analyses of the role of social media in the Arab uprisings see: www.westminster.ac.uk/__data/assets/pdf_file/0004/220675/WPCC-vol9-issue2.pdf.

References

Baars, S. and ISC (University of Manchester) (2010) Social class, aspirations and cultural capital: a case study of working class children's plans for the future and their parents' involvement in life beyond the school gates. *ISC Working Paper 2010–05* Manchester: Institute for Social Change, University of Manchester.

Beck, U. (2013) *The Digital Freedom Risk: Too Fragile an Acknowledgement*. Available at: www.opendemocracy.net/can-europe-make-it/ulrich-beck/digital-freedom-risk-too-fragile-acknowledgment.

Becker, H., Geer, B., Hughes, E.C. and Strauss, A. (1961) *Boys in White: Student Culture in Medical School*. Chicago, IL: University of Chicago Press.

Chambliss, D.F. (1996) *Beyond Caring, Hospitals, Nurses and the Social Organization of Ethics*. Chicago: Chicago University Press.

Chief Medical Officer (2001) Harold Shipman's clinical practice 1974–1998: a clinical audit commissioned by the Chief Medical Officer. London: Department of Health.

Collins, R. (1979) *The Credential Society: An Historical Sociology of Education and Stratification*. New York: Academic Press.

Cooke, H. (2012) Changing discourses of blame in nursing and healthcare. In D. Holmes, T. Rudge A. and Perron (eds) *(Re)Thinking Violence in Health Care Settings: A Critical Approach*. Farnham: Ashgate, 47–66.

Davies, C. (1995) *Gender and the Professional Predicament in Nursing*. Buckingham: Open University Press.

Davis, F. (1975) Professional socialization as a subjective experience: the process of doctrinal conversion among student nurses. In C. Cox and A. Mead (eds) *A Sociology of Medical Practice*. London: Collier-Macmillan, 116–131.

Department for Education and Skills (2005) 'Has the social class gap narrowed in primary schools?' Background note accompanying the talk by Rt Hon Ruth Kelly MP, Secretary of State for Education and Skills: 'Education and Social Progress', 26 July.

Etzioni, A. (ed.) (1969) *The Semi-Professions and Their Organization*. New York: The Free Press.

Fox, N. (2012) *The Body*. Cambridge: Polity.

Furlong, A. (1993) *Schooling for Jobs: Changes in the Career Preparation of British Secondary School Children*. Aldershot: Ashgate.

Goffman, E. (1959) *The Presentation of Self in Everyday Life*. Harmondsworth: Penguin.

Goldthorpe, J.H. (2003) The myth of education-based meritocracy: why the theory isn't working. *New Economy* 10(4): 234–239.

Guardian (2014) Christian nursery worker claims unfair dismissal over dispute with gay colleague. *Guardian*. Available at: www.theguardian.com/uk-news/2014/apr/20/christian-nursery-worker-claims-unfair-dismissal-gay-colleague (accessed 12 September 2014).

Heritage, J. (1997) Conversation analysis and institutional talk: analysing data. In D. Silverman (ed.) *Qualitative Research: Theory, Method and Practice*. London: Sage, 161–82.

Illich, I. (1977) *Medical Nemesis*. Harmondsworth: Penguin.

JM Consulting Ltd (1998) *The Regulation of Nurses, Midwives and Health Visitors; Report on a Review of the Nurses, Midwives & Health Visitors Act 1997*. Bristol: JM Consulting.

Kennedy, I. (1981) *The Unmasking of Medicine*. London: George Allen & Unwin.

Kennedy, I. and Bristol Royal Infirmary (2000) *The Inquiry into the Management of Care of Children Receiving Complex Heart Surgery at the Bristol Royal Infirmary*. Bristol: Central Office of Information.

Larson, M.S. (1977) *The Rise of Professionalism: A Sociological Analysis*. Berkeley, CA: University of California Press.

Lindsey, R.A. (2013) What the Arab Spring tells us about the future of social media in revolutionary movements. Available at: http://smallwarsjournal.com/jrnl/art/what-the-arab-spring-tells-us-about-the-future-of-social-media-in-revolutionary-movements.

Lintern, S. (2013) HEE bids to tackle staffing crisis. Available at: www.hsj.co.uk/news/exclusive-hee-bids-to-tackle-staffing-crisis/5065750.article?blocktitle=News&contentID=13251-. Uph0U6NFAdU.

Macionis, J. and Gerber, L. (2011) *Sociology*. Toronto: Pearson.

Manning, A. (2011) The successes and failures of multiculturalism. Available at: www.policy-network.net/pno_detail.aspx?ID=4084&title=The-successes-and-failures-of-multiculturalism (accessed 17 September 2014).

Mead, G. (1913) 'The social self'. *Journal of Philosophy, Psychology and Scientific Methods* 10: 374–380.

Menzies, I.E.P. (1960) A case study in the functioning of social systems as a defence against anxiety: a report on a study of the nursing service of a general hospital. *Human Relations* 13: 95–121.

Murthy, D. (2010) Towards a sociological understanding of social media: theorizing Twitter. *Sociology* 46: 1059–1073.

NANDA International (2014) *Nursing Diagnoses: Definitions and Classification 2012–2014*. Oxford: Wiley-Blackwell.

Nursing and Midwifery Council (2013) *Nursing and Midwifery Council Annual Fitness to Practise Report 2012–2013*. London: The Stationery Office.

Parsons, T. (1954) *Essays in Sociological Theory*. Glencoe: The Free Press.

Schein, E.H. (1988) Organizational socialization and the profession of management. *MIT Sloan Management Review*, 15 October. http://sloanreview.mit.edu/article/organizational-socialization-and-the-profession-of-management/ (accessed 14 September 2014).

Schultz, P.R. and Meleis, A.I. (1988) Nursing epistemology: traditions, insights, questions. *Image: the Journal of Nursing Scholarship* 20: 217–221.

Silverman, D. (1997) *Discourses of Counselling: HIV Counselling as Social Interaction*. London: Sage.

UNICEF (2007) Gender equality – the big picture. Available at: www.unicef.org/gender/index_bigpicture.html (accessed 14 September 2014)

van Dijck, J. (2013) *The Culture of Connectivity: A Critical History of Social Media*. Oxford: Oxford University Press.

Witz, A. (1992) *Professions and Patriarchy*. London: Routledge.

World Health Organization and London School of Hygeine and Tropical Medicine (2013) *Global and Regional Estimates of Violence against Women*. Geneva, Switzerland: WHO.

4

Nursing as women's work

Pam Smith and Helen Allan

Issue

The issue considered in this chapter is nursing work and how it is defined and organised. Stereotypes based on race, class and gender prevail within society and influence not only how nursing work is perceived but also the assumptions about what nurses do. Many of these stereotypes are rooted in history. When you read Chapter 5 you will see a quotation from nursing professor Sue Proctor (see page 106) who attributes the power of such stereotypes, in particular 'gender blindness', to society's failure to recognise nursing's worth and central role resulting in inequalities within the National Health Service (NHS) workforce (Proctor, 2000: 3). Global stereotypes incorporate the narratives of migration and racialisation associated with overseas trained and trainee nurses.

As you read through this chapter you will see how the issue of nursing work is closely linked to professional socialisation discussed in Chapter 3, the complex and intimate nature of care work examined in Chapters 5 and 6, and the role of management and delegation considered in Chapter 8.

This chapter brings together the sociological concepts of patriarchy, hierarchy, power and the division of labour from an historical and global perspective to analyse and reflect on the nature of nursing work and how it is valued within society in general and the healthcare workforce in particular. Patriarchy brings a wider perspective to our analysis by assisting us to understand the role of gender and stereotyping within society and its influence on the nursing profession and nursing work in terms of hierarchy, power and the division of labour, not only between doctors and nurses but also among nurses themselves. Finally, strategies adopted by nurses to confront and resist oppression are considered.

Scenario 4.1

Consider, for example, your experience as a student during clinical placements and your relationship with different members of the nursing team.

Compare your experience with the examples gathered by Pam Smith during interviews with student nurses:

A surgical ward sister was described as 'very competent, very nice, very funny. She makes the ward happy' (Smith, 1992: 77).

Another student said: 'I think students work jolly hard if they are working with someone who understands them a bit more and thanks them at the end of the shift rather than bossing them around all the time' (Smith, 1992: 79).

Students valued being treated as individuals and valuable members of the ward team.

You may have noticed that some of your clinical placement specialities are regarded as having higher status than others. For example, acute nursing is often regarded as high status work whereas care of older people is regarded as low status work.

Pam also conducted an attitude survey about the ward learning environment with first- and third-year student nurses. The scores demonstrated a pecking order of preferences with the specialist medical wards (neurology, cardiology and oncology) coming out on top and the lowest ratings being awarded to the general medical wards where the patients were elderly and suffering from chronic conditions such as chronic obstructive airways disease (COPD) and congestive cardiac failure (CCF) (Smith 1992: 53).

Note that although these findings were obtained during the 1980s they have been chosen because they reflect many of the comments made by current students. They highlight issues that we are going to discuss in the chapter about the status of different types of work and the potential role of power and hierarchy in the workplace. To what extent do you consider these examples compare with your own experiences?

Chapter outline

In this chapter we analyse nursing work through the following conceptual lenses:

• Patriarchy

We begin the chapter by exploring patriarchy, how it operates as a social system and its relationship to nursing and nurses' work. In particular we consider the definition of nurses' work as 'women's work' and the wider implications of stereotypes beyond gender, that is class and race, both historically and globally.

- Demographic characteristics, inequality and the division of labour within the healthcare workforce

We next describe the demographic characteristics of the healthcare workforce by age, gender, race and ethnicity to show their relationship to inequality within the division of labour. We present research on migrant nurses as an illustrative case study.

- Hierarchy, power and the division of labour

Hierarchy, power and the division of labour are integral to the analysis throughout the chapter and offer insights into the relationships not only between doctors and nurses but also among nurses themselves. The management and delegation of nursing work and the emergence of new nursing roles are considered.

In the final section of the chapter we consider some of the strategies nurses use to take power to resist, assert and overcome domination, oppression and scapegoating. These strategies play an important role not only when things go wrong (see Chapter 7) but also to prevent things going wrong in the first place. Strategies include joining unions, professional organisations, forming pressure groups and developing unique nursing knowledge and innovative practice such as the 'new nursing' initiatives described in Chapter 6.

Patriarchy

We begin by exploring patriarchy because it is a social system (like capitalism considered in Chapter 1) which has been hugely influential in shaping modern nursing as a gendered occupation (Walby, 1990). Like Wilkinson and Miers (1999) we agree that patriarchy affects and shapes the low status and invisibility of caring work.

Patriarchy is the social domination of women and children and younger men by older men; the recognition of men's achievements over women's. Thus nursing, historically and even today, is predominantly a female occupation, and as a result its achievements have been ignored in history (Miles, 1988) and frequently in policy; any developments in education and practice have been dominated by its relationship with medicine, or by 'medical men' (Ehrenreich and English, 1979).

Patriarchy is a social system in which: males hold primary power; males predominate in roles of political leadership, moral authority, social privilege and control of property; and, in the domain of the family, fathers or father-figures hold authority over women and children. (Walby, 1990)

Sociologist Sylvia Walby (1987) has composed six overlapping structures that define patriarchy and that take different forms in different cultures and different times:

1. The state: women are unlikely to have formal power and representation
2. The household: women are more likely to do the housework and raise the children.
3. Violence: women are more prone to being abused.
4. Paid work: women are likely to be paid less.
5. Sexuality: women's sexuality is more likely to be treated negatively.
6. Culture: women are more misrepresented in media and popular culture.

More recent work on defining patriarchy includes the observation that patriarchy is more than just the rule of individual men; it is about the rule of men through masculine institutions which hold power in societies and across societies through transglobal institutions. These institutions serve the interests and lives of men.

No analysis of women's work would be complete without reference to the feminist sociologist Ann Oakley. Oakley undertook ground-breaking research on women and housework in the 1970s when women's work was neither visible nor considered a legitimate field of study (Oakley, 1974). Many feminist scholars have followed in her wake, such as Clare Ungerson, a feminist professor of social policy who has been researching and writing about women's work for over three decades. She has repeatedly drawn attention to the dichotomy[1] between unpaid and paid care work and the private and public spaces in which it takes place (Ungerson, 1983, 2006). She suggests that women have a unique set of skills associated with their roles as mothers, many of which take place in the privacy of the home yet share much in common with 'public' institutionalised care work. Indeed, attitude surveys undertaken during the 1980s revealed that the public identified 'alertness to the needs of others' as the mark of both the good woman and the good nurse (Oakley, 1986).

Ungerson's skill set is itemised in the box below.

Reflection 4.1

(a) time available at short notice and in flexible lumps;
(b) high levels of skill in domestic tasks, e.g. cooking, cleaning, washing;
(c) high levels of social skill, such as talking and listening to assess present and future needs;
(d) skills in information gathering about other services and ability to act autonomously over a wide range of tasks of widely differing skill level;
(e) punctuality and reliability;
(f) ability to operate over long periods in fairly isolated circumstances, engaging in routine and often unpleasant tasks, particularly in the case of the very old, people with learning disabilities and mentally ill – with very little measurable 'success' or positive response from recipients.

---

[1]A dichotomy presents contrasts between two ideas – in this case the contrast between paid and unpaid care work that takes place in the public and private domains

Take a few minutes to read through Ungerson's list and, as you read, consider whether you agree with the view that these items represent the 'socially expected attributes of women' in Western Europe, but more specifically whether they apply to twenty-first-century nursing.

Recent surveys show very similar findings and a clear view that men are reluctant to work in social care because of the 'stigma' they attach to care work and its 'feminine' connotations (Lombard 2012; Franklin 2014). This is a very strong reaction indeed and Lombard poses the question of why men don't want to work in social care; you can consider whether his findings can be applied to nursing.

Reflection 4.2

The Skills for Care report on the characteristics of the social care workforce found that 82 per cent of the workforce were women and suggested that the reasons for this were that few men were attracted to work with attributes they saw as:

- equating to work with elderly people, and envisaged as being in homes;
- essentially unskilled, low paid, with flat management structures;
- a career with fairly unpleasant routine tasks.

Comparing the attributes presented first by Ungerson and then from the Skills for Care report, they appear to be very similar despite having been written 30 years apart.

In short, Lombard (2012) states: 'The social care sector has struggled to attract men to join the workforce. The "caring" occupations have been traditionally seen as female-oriented and the latest reports on the workforce show little signs of change.' Even the managers and supervisors in the sector were predominantly women at 79 per cent (this is very different to nursing where the percentage of men in management roles compared with women is high), which is a clear indicator of men's low regard of social care as a work choice (Franklin, 2014).

One of the reasons why women's skills are held in low regard is that many of the jobs they do are taken for granted. Davies[2] and Rosser (1986), in a study of women working as higher clerical officers in the health sector, introduced the term 'gendered job' to describe how gender is built into the labour process. The job draws on the

---

[2]The Davies referred to in this reference is Celia Davies, the feminist sociologist whose work on gender and nursing's 'professional predicament' was considered in Chapter 3. As you can see Davies and her co-researcher Rosser were interested in the relationship between gender and women's work more generally and not just in nursing.

qualities and capabilities women develop and acquire through the performance of their daily lives outside the workplace. But at the time that Davies and Rosser were undertaking their research, clerical officers in nursing and care work were mostly women, and the qualities and capabilities they described were regarded as part of the package rather than as an essential part of the job requiring higher status and financial rewards.

Another reason why women's work is so undervalued is because of the lack of recognition and inappropriate imposition of male notions of time on care work (Davies,[3] 1990). Flexible timetables are necessary to allow carers to respond to individuals' ever changing needs, often described as the 'little things' that may be 'difficult to capture and slip by unnoticed in the daily routines and hustle and bustle of ward life' (Smith, 1992: 1).

The 'little things' are the victims of what Davies (1990) and other writers call competing rationalities that underpin institutionalised care work. Scientific and technical-economic rationalities correspond to a male-orientated approach to care work which Davies (citing Gardell et al., 1979: 92) describes as 'assembly line care of the sick' (Davies 1990: 108). Costs are kept to a minimum and as many patients as possible are processed through medical diagnosis and treatment in the minimum time achievable. The result is that managers and accountants neither recognise nor cost the 'little things' into the work process while carers who do, struggle to 'fit them in'.

Reflection 4.3

Does this account of the work process sound familiar? Can you think of occasions when it felt like you had to work hard to 'fit in the little things' to make a difference to patients, their families and friends? These are issues that we explore further in Chapter 5.

Student work

The experience of being a student nurse has changed over time (Smith, 1992, 2012). When Pam undertook her study in the 1980s student nurses were apprentices and constituted the main workforce in the wards, giving up to 75 per cent of the direct patient care. With the introduction of supernumerary status at the beginning of the 1990s, healthcare assistants (HCAs) took over from students as the main workforce. One of their main tasks was seen as giving personal care to patients. Technical tasks became the qualified nurses' primary responsibility and a clear demarcation was made between technical and personal care.

Research with Helen (Allan et al., 2008) showed that the effect on students was complex, leading them to divide nursing work into high (technical) and low

---

[3]The Davies referred to here is Karen Davies, a Swedish researcher.

(personal) status tasks.[4] The division of tasks in this way gave students the impression that the 'hands on work' of personal care was not the 'real work' of nursing since the pressure on registered nurses to undertake the more complex technical care meant that the students rarely saw them engaged in bedside nursing. Many students resented being allocated what they saw as low status work which was often supervised by HCAs.

Tasks and targets

The organisation of the work into tasks and targets suits the busier pace of the NHS. Targets are set to process patients in under four hours through the Accident and Emergency department, manage beds to reduce hospital waiting lists and speed up discharge. More and more patients are treated as day cases for conditions such as cataracts, herniorrhaphies (hernia repairs) and cancer when in the past they might have spent weeks as inpatients. Current inpatients tend to be older, sicker and more dependent than in the past which can often mean their recovery time exceeds the discharge targets. Nurses are increasingly caught between the competing demands of technical and care work, with the inevitable loss of the 'little things' resulting in a 'care deficit' (Hochschild, 2003: 218). This means that nurses are forced to alter the care they give and clients must often learn to do without in order to meet financial targets (Bone, 2009: 57). Research in Canada has shown that such targets put undue pressure on nurses to go against their professional judgement to discharge patients because of the imperative for 'more efficient and effective use of public funds' (Rankin and Campbell, 2009: 1). This imperative resulted in systems that forced nurses to suppress their professional judgements to make decisions with negative consequences for patients (Rankin and Campbell, 2009).

Scenario 4.2

In our research the ward managers reported that their role had been affected by the target-driven nature of the NHS. The following quotation is from a ward manager who had worked as a ward sister during the 1980s. When asked how her role had changed over the years she said: 'Obviously, the NHS climate has changed since 2001. I think the target culture is here and is unavoidable. Obviously financial things, I have been much more aware than when I was a ward sister.'

(Continued)

---

[4]The division of nursing into high- and low-status tasks is a position akin to findings by Goddard (1953), Fretwell (1982), Melia (1982), Alexander (1983), Smith (1988) and Ousey (2007) spanning 60 years.

> *(Continued)*
>
> Other ward managers also said that their role had changed following the introduction of targets brought in to maintain bed occupancy and throughput in the early 2000s (DH, 2004). These trends continue and become the hallmark of successful NHS organisations but also the reasons why they fail, as in the case of the Mid-Staffordshire NHS Trust where the managers became too focused on finance at the expense of frontline care (see Chapter 7 for an analysis of when things go wrong).
>
> During an interview with a ward manager, it became clear from the following account that measures 'to increase throughput in the hospital' had had a 'frightening' effect on her: 'The priority is to increase discharges and there's no mistake made about that … to make sure discharges are going through … to increase the throughput in the hospital. And you become a sort of, I don't know, what would you call it? [The interviewee pauses to reflect before suggesting that] … You're just like an automaton. I sometimes come into the ward and I'm looking at the board in numbers and I get quite frightened sometimes because I'm forgetting [the numbers] they're people and I have to pull back.'

These accounts are living examples of how patriarchy operates through entrenched cultural beliefs based on stereotypes about femininity and masculinity (Evans, 1996) which influence the organisation of healthcare in general and nursing work in particular. We now explore these concepts further below.

Femininity and masculinity

Stereotypical beliefs about femininity are that women are nurturing, caring, subjective and less rational than men, dependent on men and submissive. These are in contrast to stereotypes about masculinity which hold that men are aggressive, strong, dominant, have self-control and objectivity.

Underpinned by these beliefs, patriarchy values and privileges the male over the female. It is important to say that patriarchy was a form of social organisation long before capitalism, but the two are deeply intertwined in industrialised societies. It is so entrenched in our thought that some societies, who recognise gender inequality and the effects this can have on women's lives (and health), have legislated against gender discrimination (UK Equality Act 2010). The recognition of the need to legislate is largely due to an important feminist critique, which we will draw on to understand and explore nursing work.

So patriarchy is a gendered social system that devalues women and women's work; we will now draw on several feminist theories to help us understand this situation. A word of caution here: feminism covers a wide range of writing and thought across disciplines outside sociology, such as psychology, anthropology and philosophy (Allan, 1993). Feminism and nursing have been discussed extensively both in sociology and nursing, and while a brief introduction is given in this section, further reading is encouraged of the references provided.

Feminism

Feminism questions principles and assumptions about gender that seem justified and part of our taken-for-granted social world (Stanley and Wise, 1993). This world is, as we have seen, patriarchal. An obvious example where sometimes assumptions go unchallenged would be in the commonly held belief that boys play with cars and girls with dolls. This seemingly *natural fact* is seen to explain these behaviours without examining the social or cultural influences that may both require boys and girls to play with different toys and seemingly predispose them to do so. This argument about boys' and girls' choices for toys is often called the nature–nurture debate.

Nursing examples may be the explanation given for why more men are nursing managers than women – are they better at being in charge or does being a male have an advantage in a female occupation? Why were men not allowed to train as health visitors until 1979? In fact, recent work suggests that small numbers of male nurses occupy a disproportionate amount of high-level managerial and speciality positions and therefore power in healthcare (Simpson, 2011; see further evidence from the King's Fund research, 2013, cited by Michael Traynor in Chapter 8 which showed women faced barriers in taking up senior NHS management and leadership roles). This has been explained by men being a) seen as high-status tokens for nursing in its relationship with medicine (Evans 1996) and b) valued and nurtured by women in the furtherance of their careers (Villeneuve 1994; Simpson 2011) or c) men do not attract the horizontal violence or oppressed group behaviour described by Street (1992).

Brooks (1997: 19) has argued that 'it is not the experience itself, but thinking from a contradictory position that produces feminist knowledge' irrespective of whether the thought is male or female. Leonardo (1991) argues that all forms of patterned inequality merit analysis in feminism. This would include therefore an analysis of social class, race and ethnicity as well as gender (see Chapter 2), and the case study of migrant nurses discussed below.

The goals of feminism are empowerment, equality and recognition of power relations in social relationships at the micro and macro levels (Letherby, 2003). The struggle for women's rights has been closely linked to struggles to establish and legitimate an educated nursing workforce (Nelson, 2010). As Nelson states: 'for nursing … to flourish, women need educational opportunities, a career path within the healthcare system and a voice in health policy and service development' (2010: 22). We only draw on a narrow range of feminist writings on professions in this section.

Patriarchy fundamentally describes *who* controls power in social relationships and societies – older men – *over whom* – women, children and younger men. We shall now consider the sociological explanations to the following questions: Do men control nursing and if they do, why? Do men control nursing because at the time nursing as a profession in the West began to establish itself, nurses were women and doctors were men?

The gendered division of labour

Feminist sociologists certainly think so. Sociologists like Sylvia Walby (1987), Ann Witz (1990), Celia Davies (1995), whom we refer to above and in Chapter 3, have explained nursing's position as an occupation or a semi-profession rather than a profession by the gendered division of labour[5] in healthcare. By this we mean that women and men have tended to be recruited and *self*-recruit into occupations and professions in a predictable gendered pattern (Warwick-Booth, 2013). Connell (2009) suggests that as globalism now dominates business, trade and other areas of work, so the gendered division of labour and gender relations are globalised to the benefit of men; that is, transnational companies and non-governmental agencies like the United Nations and the World Health Organization tend to have male managers and the international media tend to report a male view of global issues such as migration and ignore women's issues.

But the gendered division of labour is more than the recruitment of men and women into different occupations or professions because, as we have said, nursing and medicine are not equal professions in the UK or anywhere really. So any discussion of the gendered division of labour must consider: 1) how each profession either assumes the characteristics of the dominant gender in that occupation or recruits to meet those gender characteristics; and 2) how the work that each occupation does is valued in society.

The characteristics associated with masculinity and femininity described above tend to be seen as natural explanations for men and women's occupational roles (Warwick-Booth, 2013). This is particularly strong for nursing where nursing tasks were similar to nineteenth-century domestic tasks which were seen as low skill in comparison with emerging industrial skills and, as a consequence, were devalued. Porter (1992) calls this *the patriarchal feminine* which values the masculine role above the feminine. It is also a good example of the complex ways in which capitalism built on existing oppressive structures in patriarchy.

The labour market is more recently thought of as increasingly feminised, that is with more women in the labour market, which has tended to deconstruct the gendered nature of work (Simpson, 2011). As agents, individuals may challenge dominant notions of gender. Yet as Martin (2006) argues, sociologists have yet to really show this consistently or understand how individuals and groups engage with dominant gender stereotypes in such strongly gendered occupations such as nursing. Feminist sociologists have argued that such readings of the power of the individual to reflexively challenge and shape gender in work overestimates the power of the individual to effectively change social structures. Simpson (2011: 387) concludes that in nursing, while female nurses might bemoan 'men's tendency to leave the dirty work of nursing to women, they frequently drew on traditionally gendered justificatory logic to explain these behaviours'; in other words, the women nurses reverted to explaining men's tendency to avoid dirty work by saying they were better at decision-making and leadership. As one male nurse from Simpson's study explained the different positions of men and women in the nursing hierarchy: 'women are just more emotional … more emotionally tied to their patients' (2011: 389).

---

[5]The phrase sexual division of labour refers to the division of labour within the family based on men and women's sexual roles in the family, effectively women's childbearing and breast-feeding roles. The gendered division of labour refers to roles outside the home in the developing capitalist system in the eighteenth and nineteenth centuries.

However, as our research accounts illustrate (Allan et al., 2008), scientific and technical-economic rationalities akin to male-orientated 'assembly line care of the sick' which underpin target-driven healthcare, create tensions, divisions and internal hierarchies between registered nurses, students and healthcare assistants, and shape their perceptions of the relative status between technical and personal nursing care.

Sexual orientation

Sexual orientation is an important dimension of nursing as gendered work and has been the subject of study by a number of authors (Platzer, 1988; Clarke, 2014). Clarke's thesis (2014) explores how gay student nurses negotiate their gender, masculinity and gay sexuality within the professional boundaries of nursing. The theoretical framing of the thesis draws upon Goffman's theories of presentation and performance of the self (Goffman, 1956).

Furthermore, it identifies how these students negotiate issues of caring and the formation of therapeutic relationships with their patients, as men and gay men. It examines their 'fraught and precarious' negotiation of the nursing role as gay men associated with the complexities and boundaries of professional nursing roles in contemporary healthcare. In particular, Clarke explores the portrayal of nursing work as mothering, nurturing and caring, which he sees as problematic because not all women necessarily possess these qualities, while many men do. Assigning women these traditional roles reinforces women's powerless position. Furthermore, stereotyping gay men as caring (and also effeminate) further emphasises women's (as well as nurses' and gay male nurses') subordinate position within patriarchal society. Through in-depth interviews with gay student nurses Clarke was able to move away from stereotypical notions of caring towards an understanding of each participant's personal narrative. He also considers the implications of his findings for lesbian, bisexual and transgender nurses.[6]

Nursing as low-paid women's work

Gender has also played a significant part in unequal pay between men and women and nurses have been regarded as underpaid for their work. This is a problem generally attributed to the predominance of women within the profession and to a middle-class vocationally orientated leadership (Abel-Smith, 1960; Carpenter, 1977; Davies, 1980).

However, during the 1960s, increasing numbers of men in general nursing and mental health raised their profile in unions and professional organisations and the new managerial hierarchies. The result was a gender hierarchy within the profession: by the 1980s men formed about 10 per cent of the nursing workforce but occupied 50 per cent of the management positions – a situation that continues in the 2000s (Whittock et al., 2002). Rates of pay subsequently improved, particularly for those in managerial and specialist nurse posts.

---

[6] The invisibility of lesbian nurses in the literature is striking. Robertson (1992) described them as 'an invisible minority' a view confirmed by Rose (1993) and elaborated by Randal and Eliason (2012).

Current rates show that the top-of-the-scale nurse consultants and managers can earn up to £65,922, with the highest salary topping £77,850 (pay rates 2015–16, RCN). The minimum starting salary for a registered nurse is £21,692, increasing to £31,072 for a senior staff or charge nurse (pay rates 2015–16, RCN). Care assistants earn between £15,100 and £16,633 (pay rates 2015–16, RCN). The pay differential between the different grades is very marked. Social care work is considerably less well remunerated and there is evidence of private employers exploiting workers by not paying them the national minimum wage of £6.70 (2015) per hour (Low Pay Commission, 2013; Franklin, 2014)

Reflection 4.4

Here are two websites for you to investigate the salary scales of different grades of nurses but also other healthcare professionals working in the NHS so you will be able to compare and contrast how different types of work are remunerated and by implication valued.

www.nhscareers.nhs.uk/explore-by-career/nursing/pay-for-nurses

www.rcn.org.uk/employment-and-pay/nhs-pay-scales-2015-16

The gendered division of labour has begun to change in medicine, where 50 per cent of medical college recruits are women; yet in more high-status specialities of medicine, men tend to be more prominent. So a gendered division of labour can exist at entry points to an occupation and at promotion points within an occupation. Women continue to be the majority in nursing, with 10 per cent of nurses being male (NMC, 2011). This 10 per cent has remained remarkably consistent over many years but with more men being in management positions (see above and Chapter 8). However, while in the 1980s, there was a concerted effort to recruit more women into medicine, there has never been a similar strategy in nursing to increase the intake of men. Nursing remains a female-dominated occupation that has developed without the professional status accorded to medicine. So where do these gender stereotypes come from? Many of them are rooted in history.

Lessons from history

Modern UK nursing traces its origins to Victorian Britain and the powerful image of Florence Nightingale. Nightingale set up the first formal nursing school in Britain at St Thomas' voluntary hospital in London. According to Abel-Smith[7] (1960) the voluntary hospitals (the forerunners of the 'high-status' teaching hospitals) provided a suitable occupation for the daughters of the Victorian upper social classes (Abel-Smith, 1960).

---

[7]Brian Abel-Smith (1926–1996) was a British economist and expert adviser who was influential in shaping twentieth-century health and social welfare.

Nursing was seen as a 'vocation' and its characteristics the epitome of the 'good' woman, requiring duty, devotion and obedience. A *Daily Telegraph* correspondent writing in 1888 stated quite categorically that 'No sensible woman objects to acknowledging what is the fact, that she is physically and intellectually inferior to men'. In other words women were expected to behave in keeping with Victorian middle-class social values by recognising their inferiority to men. The inference for the emerging nursing profession was that nurses (women) were expected to be subordinate to doctors (men).

Gamarnikov (1978) has written that the early relationship between doctors and nurses was based on the Victorian family model: the doctor was the father, the nurse the mother and the patient the child. In other words, the nurse–doctor–patient relationship mirrors the power relations between men, women and children within the patriarchal family.

Carpenter (1978) links this model to the reproduction of the wider Victorian class structure based not only on preconceived notions of the division of labour between the sexes (male doctors and female nurses) but also class (upper-class matrons and ward sisters; lower-class nurses and domestic servants). To paraphrase Carpenter's interpretation of this family model:

> The ward sister or matron complemented the authority of the doctor (a man) in organising the nurses and domestic staff in a mirror image of how, as the 'lady of the house', she would have supported her husband and supervised the servants.

In terms of social class, Nightingale's role in the shaping of modern nursing has been seen as a response to the need to create a respectable profession for a surplus of upper-middle-class women in the mid-nineteenth century. Nursing became that respectable profession but from early on was dominated by a class hierarchy reflected in nurses' positions and locations. A model of nurse training was developed in the élite[8] voluntary hospitals to train matrons as leaders of bedside nurses. In Carpenter's view this model came about because care work was regarded as lower class but 'carried out under the moral leadership of upper class women' (1977: 168).

Matrons were recruited to manage and organise the nursing workforce to deliver frontline care in the poor-law institutions, predominantly staffed by working-class female nurses and the large mental hospitals or asylums, which traditionally recruited working-class men (Abel-Smith, 1960; Davies, 1980). These institutions came to be associated with a 'pecking order' of medically defined specialties. The voluntary (future teaching) hospitals, through their association with acute illness, later provided the foundation for prestigious 'high-tech' care rather than the 'routine and basic' care provided by the poor-law institutions and asylums for the elderly and the mentally and chronically ill. By the beginning of the twentieth century an overall association between class and prestigious positions within nursing located within the elite voluntary hospitals had been established. Working-class nurses of both genders working in the poor-law institutions and asylums remained on the margins (Davies, 1980). On the basis of this evidence, Carpenter concludes that 'sex, class and later racial insignia were attached to the division of labour as the basis for hospital stratification' (1977: 168).

'Racial insignia' did not play an explicit role in the creation of nursing divisions and disadvantage until the first wave of migration following the Second World War. However,

---

[8]Merton's (1948/1968) theory of elites is relevant here. He points out that elites may use their power over others for their own benefit but with detrimental effects on other groups.

Seacole's story is a clear example of how the early nursing elite marginalised and devalued skills and expertise based on race and class (Alexander and Dewjee, 1984; Smith, 1987).

Here are two scenarios that present different and alternative images of iconic nurses from history. The first is Mary Seacole who was a contemporary of Florence Nightingale and equally famous in her day.

Scenario 4.3   Mary Seacole

Mary Seacole, a Jamaican-Scottish healer, herbalist and businesswoman once shunned by Florence Nightingale and the Victorian establishment, has risen to prominence to take her rightful place in nursing history. Until the 1980s her story was little known and in many ways epitomised the marginalisation and devaluation that black nurses subsequently experienced (Alexander and Dewjee, 1984; Smith, 1987; Baxter, 1988, Smith and Mackintosh, 2007). Seacole, who was well established in Jamaica, regarded it her duty as a loyal citizen of the British Empire to travel to London to offer her services as a nurse in the Crimean War. Although her offer was rejected she used her own means to travel to the war zone and care for injured and dying soldiers. She returned to the UK almost penniless but a group of grateful soldiers organised a concert to raise funds for her. There are now portraits of Seacole to be seen in the National Portrait Gallery and the Royal College of Nursing in London which testify to the work undertaken by the Jamaican Nurses' Association and the annual Black History month which over the past 30 years has highlighted the achievements of Seacole and other prominent members of the black community to reveal their hidden history.

The second is iconic Islamic nurse Hazrat Zainab who was the first granddaughter of the Prophet Mohammed and, in this scenario, a role model to contemporary Islamic student nurses.

Scenario 4.4   Hazrat Zainab

Read the extract from the thesis of one of our doctoral students who was researching the experiences of student nurses in Saudi Arabia and their decision to continue or leave nursing (Alfaraj, 2008):

One student nurse explained explicitly how she took Prophet Mohammed's granddaughter Hazrat Zainab as an idol to ease her frustration caused by joining nursing. This student nurse believed that nursing was the occupation decided for her by God and because the Prophet's granddaughter nursed wounded and ill people during her time; therefore the student nurse thought that by following the actions of the Prophet's granddaughter and God's will her own misery would be alleviated.

The student nurse was seen as a deviant case because her coping mechanism to deal with the difficulties during pre-clinical exposure was linked to her religious beliefs; that is, she would be rewarded later by God because of her suffering.

As the influence of Islam and other societies becomes more and more prominent it is important to consider the role of nursing in different historical, cultural and religious contexts. Reflect on the stories of Mary Seacole and Hazrat Zainab and the lessons to be learned from their lives as nurses and their work in war zones.

As we can see above and from the different images and activities that come to mind, nursing is not a homogeneous profession and the work is diverse.

A quick look at the NHS nursing careers website confirms this, with 32 different categories of nurse, specialist nurse, health visitor, team manager in hospital and community specified: www.nhscareers.nhs.uk/explore-by-career/nursing/.

History and hierarchies

History reveals a constant making and remaking of hierarchy and division both as a professionalising strategy and to deliver hands-on care. That professional hierarchies are structured in part on social divisions of class, gender and race is a constant of British nursing experience. These divisions are played out through different types of education, management structures, institutional hierarchies and behaviour, and the pecking order of specialities (Smith and Mackintosh, 2007).

These origins go some way to explaining why nursing has still not been accorded full professional status. As we saw in Chapter 3, professional status carries with it certain advantages, one of which is the power to determine what the professional does at work. However, as we shall see, nursing work has historically been difficult to define because it is assumed to be women's 'natural' work and is devalued compared with other healthcare work.

Scenario 4.5

In 2011 the British newspaper the *Daily Mail* cited Dr Peter Carter the general secretary of the Royal College of Nursing as saying:

Trainee nurses 'spend too long in lecture halls and not enough time with patients'... Dr Carter also warned that untrained healthcare assistants now carry out many tasks once reserved for nurses. (Borland, 2011)

(Continued)

(Continued)

The coverage provoked strong reactions. One nurse commented: 'This isn't 1911- nurses don't just prance around, mopping fevered foreheads and giving bed baths. They do that on top of the fact they are responsible for administering drugs, including IV medications that can be very complex to work out the correct doses and work complex technology vital to patient care'.

An NHS cancer patient made similar comments: 'I have been well treated by almost all staff especially nurses ... I was surprised at how much technology nurses now have to deal with and how complex some of it is. They are knowledgeable about equipment and treatment and usually very willing to explain. Clearly (the two) hospitals have training and procedures which encourage nurses to engage with patients and be responsive'.

These descriptions highlight the different aspects of nursing work involving technical, physical and emotional skills in order to ensure holistic care. But as the research examples quoted above illustrate, inherent tensions remain in how modern nursing and skills are recognised and valued.

Freidson (1970) suggests that nurses can never be completely professionally autonomous, because traditionally their knowledge and skills revolve around the diagnostic and treatment model of care. This view is apparent in Scenario 4.5 above where the nurse is portrayed as taking responsibility for treatments and medications (primarily prescribed by doctors) to ensure they are administered correctly. It is not surprising therefore that in the public's eyes nurses are often seen as doctors' assistants. They also rely on being part of the medical division of labour for their claims to being professional, as was discussed in some detail in Chapter 3. Nurses are seeking their own knowledge base and work methods based on alternative paradigms of healing, holism and emotional care in order to free themselves from medical dominance as discussed in Chapters 5 and 6. In Chapter 8 you will encounter the sociological concepts of 'gender' and 'division of labour' again in relation to 'leadership and management' but also 'managerialism'.

In order to contribute further to your sociological understanding of 'managerialism' we introduce you to a discussion by Mick Carpenter (1977, 1978) who uses the concept to show how the introduction of nurse managers has emphasised an internal hierarchy and division of labour within the nursing workforce that affords high-status, value and prestige to administrative work alongside technical tasks and over and above personal care work. The introduction of 'managerialism' to the work process can be seen therefore as a professionalising strategy within nursing to gain more status and control.

A more recent version of the internal hierarchy is the introduction of healthcare assistants to replace students as the main workforce to undertake patients' personal care, regarded as lower-status work. The impact on the division of labour between different levels of nurses and healthcare assistants is discussed in some detail by Michael in Chapter 8.

Michael undertook a study of community nursing in the 1990s which showed how 'managerialism' was influenced by 'Thatcherism',[9] the main political driver of the day (Traynor, 1999). There was a shift in the provision of health and social services from the state to the market, requiring fierce cutbacks, euphemistically referred to as 'meeting financial targets' and 'efficiency savings'. There was a subsequent loss of services that affected the relationships between managers and frontline practitioners because of the differences in their aspirations and goals. Managers were committed to cutbacks while frontline providers such as district nurses found they no longer had control over the essential resources they needed to provide an acceptable level of quality care to highly dependent patients.

The following conversations provide examples of the competing values and perceptions expressed by 'rational' managers who wished to re-organise the work in terms of saving money and district nurses committed to working to provide an acceptable level of care for patients whatever the personal costs to themselves.

Scenario 4.6

One district nurse described her work 'as a constant battle against the clock. My patients only receive the care they need because I stay late and miss lunch hours to get my paperwork done.' Managers on the other hand described the nurses as 'headless chickens' who were over-involved with their patients and needed to be more rational in their priority setting and decision-making to meet the new targets.

Race, class and gender: the case of migrant nurses

The experiences of racism and exploitation of recently arrived overseas nurses in the 2000s from both European Union (EU), non-EU and Commonwealth countries recalls experiences of an earlier generation of migrant nurses from Ireland and the Caribbean. The nursing labour market displays sharp segmentation (in the economic sense) into more privileged and stable segments of the profession as compared with much lower paid segments with poorer working conditions. Professional restructuring has interacted with privatisation in the healthcare and social care sector, notably the private provision of nursing and residential care, to harden these inequalities. This process in turn has been facilitated by a sharp rise in migration to the UK of internationally qualified professional nurses. Research shows that the managerial reforms of healthcare and social care have tended systematically to disadvantage lower-paid, largely

---

[9]Thatcherism describes the conviction politics, socioeconomic policy and political style of the British Conservative politician Margaret Thatcher, who was leader of her party from 1975 to 1990 and prime minster from 1979 to 1990 (Gamble, 1988; Vinen, 2009). Thatcher changed Britain, irrevocably. She featured in many controversial actions, from stopping free school milk in September 1971 to breaking the bitter miners' strike (1984–85) (Beckett and Hencke 2009; Holden 2005).

female staff who care for some of the most disadvantaged members of the population (Towers et al., 1999; Smith et al., 1993). A recent survey shows similar trends in the social care sector, where black and minority ethnic groups account for 17.8 per cent of the total workforce. The sector is also reliant on non-British workers, with 18.2 per cent of the workforce accounted for by non-British workers, though managers are significantly more likely to be British (92.4 per cent) (Franklin, 2014).

Until the 1950s Baxter (1988) found that hospitals relied on Irish workers and that a drop in Irish migrants redirected recruitment campaigns towards the Commonwealth countries. Immigration policies were relaxed to allow a steady supply of trainee nurses from overseas until the 1970s, supported by common nursing curricula within the Commonwealth. Overseas nurses reached a peak in 1970 and declined considerably thereafter (Stalker, 2000). In particular, black nurse recruits fell from 10,556 in 1972 to 6,597 in 1976 (Pearson, 1985).

By 1977 12 per cent of student nurses and midwives were from overseas (66 per cent from the New Commonwealth and 22 per cent from Ireland). Twenty-one per cent of the New Commonwealth student nurses came from Malaysia, 15 per cent from the West Indies and 8 per cent from Mauritius (Doyal et al., 1980).

Baxter (1988) cites evidence that overseas nurses were located in the less prestigious institutions, specialities and lower grades of nursing. Only 7 per cent of the overseas student midwives and nurses were studying in the well-known London teaching hospitals (Doyal et al., 1980). Some new recruits are known to have been directed to undertake enrolled nurse training,[10] unaware that there were two training routes with different career opportunities (Hardill and Macdonald, 2000: 684).

Baxter (1988) described racism as a major but under-reported feature of overseas nurses' experiences of working in the health service and one of the reasons why she suggested they could become 'an endangered species' given their subsequent low recruitment rates.

As part of general disinvestment in the NHS in the 1980s, there was a huge drop in nurse education in the UK. Wages and conditions declined relative to other professions, and a drop in arrivals of migrant nurses occurred in the early 1990s, when nursing lost its designation as a 'shortage' profession (Seccombe and Ball, 1992). In addition, the 1980s saw a switch to private provision of long-term care – and the rise of private payment for such care – implying a higher proportion of recruitment undertaken by private employers.

By the time demand for nurses in high-income countries rose sharply again in the 1990s, a number of structures were in place to support a sharp rise in migration, including the 'internationalisation of nursing', cross-boundary recognition of qualifications within the EU and the development of higher education as an export business to attract overseas recruits (Iredale, 2001; Adhikari, 2010). Changes in policy and visa systems in the USA, UK and Japan and inter-governmental agreements, encouraged recruiting. These were met by a rise in international professional migration underpinned by commercial investment in labour-market movement – the 'trade of nurses' as one researcher calls it (Ball, 2004). The international labour market became much more integrated as migration was facilitated through

---

[10]Enrolled nurse training was introduced following the Second World War and phased out in the 1980s. It was a two-year programme with limited career prospects.

commercialisation of the hiring process by employment agencies, and technological and social changes greatly increased access to information (Adhikari, 2010).

The NHS Plan for 2000 set out ambitious targets for increasing the workforce and active recruitment of overseas nurses was a key strategy. In the seven years to March 2005, over 71,000 nurses educated outside the UK registered with the Nursing and Midwifery Council (NMC), representing 37 per cent of all new registrants (NMC, 2005). Total new registrations climbed fast from 1998/99, and most of the increase was initially constituted by registrations of nurses educated outside the EU. By 2005, although overseas registrations had fallen slightly, they remained high at over 11,000 per annum (NMC, 2005). However, in 2006 the UK government removed nursing from the list of shortage occupations reversing the trend until the present. As of November 2015 nursing is back on the list: www.gov.uk/government/publications/tier-2-shortage-occupation-list.

Migration now

A recent headline in the *Guardian* newspaper reads: 'New immigration rules will cost the NHS millions, warns nursing unions' (Siddique, 2015).

New immigration rules have been introduced with effect from April 2016 which mean that any non-EU worker who has been in the UK for six years will be deported if they are earning less than £35,000. As you can see from nurses' average pay rates this means that many non-EU nurses will be at risk, causing chaos within the NHS and social care sector. The Royal College of Nursing (RCN) has spoken out requesting the Home Office to add nurses to the list of shortage occupations with obvious effect (see above).

You can read further at: www.theguardian.com/society/2015/jun/22/new-immigration-rules-cost-nhs-millions-nursing.

As you can see from this account, the nursing workforce becomes a political and economic football at the mercy of the market and lower pay because of a combination of factors such as gender, class, race and ethnicity.

The interaction of hierarchy, race and ethnicity in the workplace

The following accounts are taken from a study we conducted with colleagues during 2005–2006 when the recruitment of overseas nurses was at its height and about to be taken off the list of shortage occupations (Smith et al., 2006). The research brought important insights about the experience of overseas nurses from different countries. We have selected data extracts that demonstrate the complex relationships between different groups which go beyond issues of race and skin colour, shaped by organisational cultures, structures and practices. In particular the extracts demonstrate the interaction amongst a range of ethnic groups which are framed by their position in a post-colonial hierarchy of ethnicities within the NHS.

One Ghanaian nurse expressed solidarity with African Caribbeans regarding them as 'one people': 'I think I have a very good relationship with the [Jamaicans] on my ward. I think we see ourselves as one people.' Other African nurses said that when they first arrived in the UK they were mentored by African Caribbean nurses who taught them how to adapt to the NHS by being more assertive. One nurse described her relationships with African Caribbean nurses in her first post as follows: 'We speak [quietly] … I found it challenging, but they helped me talk more as I was very quiet. So I always say I am glad I worked there first as they made me stronger.' The quote below demonstrates the construction of professional ethnic hierarchies in the NHS based on colonial hierarchies. An African Caribbean informant captures the essence of this hierarchy:

> People say that there is a pecking order in the NHS to get positions. So it's White first, White British first, then White Australian, White South African. When you run out of all of that and you have only got Black left after all the Whites its Asians. After the Asians you come down to Black and if you have to differentiate it's Black Caribbean then Black African … It's a pecking order.

The same informant went on to link the position in the hierarchy to cultural skills and acceptability of different cultures:

> I think that a lot of the Black Africans feel that in the pecking order the Caribbean will come first and I think that is probably true. I think that is true because Black Caribbeans understand British culture and how it works because a lot of us have come from British colonies. We have learned how to deal with and what to say and how to say it and I think because of that we have a little bit of advantage.

The insights offered by these research findings are important on several levels. Overall, the importance of cultural skills and proximity to the dominant cultures in navigating the workplace and in the different ways people interpret experiences in the workplace are highlighted. Thus African Caribbeans are more likely to understand processes in the UK workplace because they are more familiar with them than African nurses.

In London and other urban areas, the historical presence of African Caribbean communities and particularly nurses with histories of cultural exchange make African Caribbeans closer to the dominant communities in terms of culture and language. This is evident from another quote from the same source:

> The British White population [are] on the side of the Caribbeans more. I think that people want to work with who they are comfortable with and I think that the British are not are not as comfortable with Black Africans as they are with Black Caribbeans. So they prefer to go with those they feel more comfortable with and who they understand. Whereas I think that they feel that they don't understand the Black Africans.

However, as a Ghanaian midwife noted, although there was improved mobility among African Caribbeans relative to Africans, which she attributed to their familiarity with the system, there were still limitations to them rising in the hierarchy: 'The West Indians have done a little bit better [than Africans] … But even then I haven't seen that many that have gone that high.'

Critically, one of the informants also points to the post-colonial power relationships that underpin the construction of the hierarchy which frames the workplace interactions of African and African Caribbean nurses and midwives. These hierarchies are a legacy of colonialism and are underpinned by the cultural power of dominant ethnicities to decide who is a stranger and treat them as an outsider.

Taking power

In this chapter we have brought together the sociological concepts of patriarchy, hierarchy, power and the division of labour, taking a broad-brush approach from an historical, contemporary and global perspective. Our aim was to assist you to navigate your way through the complex world of studying and working in nursing to analyse and reflect on the nature of nursing work and how it is valued within society in general and the healthcare workforce in particular. Patriarchy brings a wider perspective to our analysis by assisting us to understand the role of gender, race, class and stereotyping within society to influence the world of work as an individual professional and through our relationships and power relations with others in the healthcare team. Life as a nurse isn't always easy. Sometimes we come up against situations and values that we don't always agree with or understand, where we are dependent on maintaining good relations with people both junior and senior to ourselves from a variety of backgrounds. It is important therefore that we make an effort to understand some of the factors that 'make people tick' and where they are coming from. This is particularly important at this moment in history where the conflicts and wars in the Middle East and Africa have triggered an exodus of traumatised migrants and refugees fleeing to Europe. It is most important that we maintain an open mind and a capacity to understand what it is like to be 'other', different to ourselves. This chapter has introduced you to some of the factors that need to be considered as well as assisting you to reflect on your own role in workplace relations.

Given the complex and demanding nature of nursing work we introduce you to some strategies adopted by nurses to confront and resist oppression. During the 1980s Pam was a member of a pressure group called Radical Nurses. Jane Salvage's book *Politics of Nursing* came out of the conversations, conferences, meetings and workshops generated by the group linked by networks across the UK (Salvage, 1985). Many of the core members had been exposed to influences such as going to university, in contrast to the pre-Project 2000 days when students learned on the job as apprentices and only a handful had been engaged in higher education[11] and/or engaged as union activists. During the 1970s and 1980s the unions were strong. We have already mentioned Prime Minister Margaret Thatcher in terms of the measures she introduced to curtail the role of the state in health, welfare, education and housing by introducing privatisation, and curbing the professions and the labour movement, epitomised by the miners' strike. The aftermath of the miners' strike saw the end of coal mining as a major British industry and the weakening of the trade-union movement generally.

However, a number of trade unions and professional organisations continue to serve health and social service employees, available to students, healthcare assistants and nurses.

The unions and professional organisations are committed to supporting their members to maintain a satisfactory work–life balance and defending rights, promoting anti-discriminatory practices and promoting health and safety in the workplace. The history of the trade-union movement is very important and played a key role in establishing the UK National Health Service in 1948. One of the ongoing roles a union can play is in supporting its members to take industrial action and withdraw their labour

---

[11]This usually meant that nurses had either taken a degree before or after qualifying as a nurse. Only a very few nurses at that time read nursing directly as a university subject at the Universities of Edinburgh, Manchester, Southampton, Surrey and King's College London.

if the need arises. The RCN, which is primarily a professional organisation, has been reluctant to support strike action, although in May 2015 when the newly elected Conservative government under David Cameron was pledging to introduce a seven-day working week in the NHS at the same time as cutting the extra pay due for working unsocial hours, the RCN stepped in at this point alongside Unite and UNISON to threaten strike action if these plans continued (Cooper and McSmith, 2015).

The RCN and the unions have an interesting history and, as mentioned above, represented different types of nurses reflected in their class, gender, race and ethnicity. If you wish to know more about this fascinating history you can read feminist and sociologist Celia Davies' edited book, referred to above, in which she revisits nursing history to include not only the Victorian middle-class ladies in the voluntary hospitals but also the men and some women working in the then-styled lunatic asylums and former workhouses (Davies, 1980). There was a growth of healthcare unions in the asylums and workhouses. Many community nurses have subsequently aligned with the unions rather than the RCN. The Unite union, for example, hosts the Health Visitors' and School Nurses' Associations. Nurses working in universities often join the RCN and the university and college union. As a student you will be entitled to be a member of your university's student union.

The history of unions, nurses' associations and strike action is very prominent in the USA. The literature is littered with reports of nurses taking action to defend their own and patients' benefits in a country that does not have a national health service and where there has been strong opposition on the part of the Republicans, the insurance companies and the multinational pharmaceutical companies to Clinton's health reforms in the 1990s and more recently with the introduction of ObamaCare. An article entitled 'Largest ever nurses' strike' (Lowes, 2010), talking about a strike involving such organisations as the California Nurses' Association and National Nurses United declared that they would take 'action whenever hospitals put profits above patient care and the wellbeing of nurses'. This is interesting in relation to our discussion above where nursing and care work get constrained by hitting financial targets, turning patients into numbers rather than holistic individuals.

Scenario 4.7   Unions and professional organisations

It is worth finding out what the different unions and professional organisations have to offer.

The RCN, for example, recently organised a job fair entitled 'Work to live or live to work'. The fair promised to help attendees find their 'dream job', hallmarks of which were: improving work/life balance, getting a well-deserved pay rise or even decreasing their commute. It is useful for you to think what you want to get from being a nurse, what indeed would be your 'perfect job'.

The RCN with 420,000 nurse and midwife members promises to 'represent, support and protect, develop, build'. UNISON, with nearly half a million members who work in the NHS, declares: 'We recognise and defend the rights of all workers in the health service. By working together within UNISON, health sector workers are better able to fight for change.' Unite the Union's main web page encourages people to join a 'structure based around the industries members work in and the regions where they love. This ensures every member gets the best representation at local and national level.'

The unions and professional organisations are all committed to defending their members against discrimination in the workplace, to address issues raised in this chapter, fighting for their rights and preventing exploitation.

Visiting the websites of the different organisations will give you a flavour of what they claim they will do for you. They all have a separate student membership and reduced fee.

Chapter summary

Whichever form of support you choose, the purpose of this chapter has been to provide you with a sociological understanding of work, how it is structured and organised to open up a world of possibilities as you embark on your chosen career. Scenarios and reflections have been provided to give you the opportunity to explore a wide range of sociological concepts and demographic factors from research, history and policy to apply them to practice.

Going further

Classic research texts

Alexander, M.F. (1983) *Learning to Nurse*. Edinburgh: Churchill Livingstone.

Goddard, H.A. (1953) *The Work of Nurses in Hospital Wards: Report of a Job Analysis*. Oxford: Nuffield Provincial Hospitals Trust.

Fretwell, J.E. (1982) *Ward Teaching and Learning: Sister and the Learning Environment*. London: Royal College of Nursing.

Melia, K.M. (1982) 'Tell it as it is' – qualitative methodology and nursing research: understanding the student nurses' world. *Journal of Advanced Nursing* 7: 327–35.

Ousey, K. (2007) Being a real nurse: nurses accounts of learning and working in practice. PhD thesis, University of Salford.

Smith, P.A. (1988) Quality of nursing and the ward as a learning environment for student nurses. PhD thesis, London: King's College, University of London.

Lesbian nurses

Robertson, M.M. (1992) Lesbians as an invisible minority in the health services arena. *Health Care for Women International* 13(2): 155–163.

Rose, P. (1993) Out in the open? *Lesbianism. Nursing Times* 89: 30, 50–5.

References

Abel-Smith, B. (1960) *A History of the Nursing Profession*. London: Heinemann.

Adhikari, R. (2010) 'The dream trap'. Brokering 'study abroad' and nurse migration from Nepal to the UK. *European Bulletin for Himalayan Research* 35–36, Autumn 2009– Spring 2010 Special Double Issue: Nepalese Migration.

Alfaraj, E. (2008) Experiences of student nurses in Saudi Arabia: the impact of clinical exposure on their decision to continue or leave nursing. PhD thesis, University of Surrey.

Alexander, Z. and Dewjee, A. (eds) (1984) *The Wonderful Adventures of Mrs Seacole in Many Lands*. Bristol: Falling Wall Press.

Allan, H.T. (1993) Feminism: a concept analysis. *Journal of Advanced Nursing* 18: 1547–1553.

Allan, H., Smith, P., Lorentzon, M. and O'Driscoll, M. (2008) *Leadership for Learning*. Report to the General Nursing Council Trust.

Ball, R.B. (2004) Divergent development, racialised rights: globalised labour markets and the trade of nurses – the case of the Philippines. *Women's Studies International Forum* 27: 119–133.

Baxter, C. (1988) The Black Nurse: *An Endangered Species*, Cambridge, National Extension College for Race and Health

Beckett, F. and Hencke, D. (2009) *Marching to the Fault Line: The Miners' Strike and the Battle for Industrial Britain*. London: Constable.

Bone, D. (2009) Epidurals not emotions: the care deficit in US maternity care. In B. Hunter and R. Deery (eds) *Emotions in Midwifery and Reproduction*. Basingstoke: Palgrave Macmillan, pp. 56–72.

Borland S (2011) Trainee nurses 'spend too long in lecture halls and not enough time with patients'. *Daily Mail*, 23 September. Available at: www.dailymail.co.uk/health/article-2040825/Trainee-nurses-spend-time-patients.html (accessed 6 November 2015).

Brooks, A. (1997) *PostFeminisms, Feminism, Cultural Theory and Cultural Forms*. London: Routledge.

Carpenter, M. (1977) The new managerialism and professionalism in nursing. In M. Stacey, M. Reid, C. Heath and R. Dingwall (eds) *Health and the Division of Labour*. London: Croom Helm.

Carpenter, M. (1978) Managerialism and the division of labour in nursing. In R. Dingwall and J. Mcintosh (eds) *Readings in the Sociology of Nursing*. Edinburgh: Churchill Livingstone.

Clarke, D. (2014) The experience of gay male undergraduate nursing students: a qualitative exploration of professional lives. PhD thesis, Cardiff University.

Connell, R.W. (2009) *Gender: In World Perspective*. Cambridge: Polity Press.

Cooper, C. and McSmith, A. (2015) Nurses may call strike if government tries to cut pay as David Cameron vows to deliver 'truly seven-day NHS' plans. *Independent*, 18 May. Available at: www.independent.co.uk/life-style/health-and-families/health-news/nurses-may-call-strike-over-plans-for-truly-sevenday-nhs-10256874.html (accessed 2 September 2015).

Davies, C. (ed.) (1980) *Rewriting Nursing History*. London: Croom Helm.

Davies, C. (1995) *Gender and the Professional Predicament of Nursing*. Buckingham: Open University Press.

Davies, C. and Rosser, J. (1986) Gendered jobs in the health service: a problem for labour process analysis. In D. Knights and H. Wilmott (eds) *Gender and the Labour Process*. Aldershot: Gower.

Davies, K. (1990) *Women and Time: Weaving the Strands of Everyday Life*. Aldershot: Avebury.

Department of Health (DH) (2004) *National Standards, Local Action: Health and Social Care Standards and Planning Framework 2005/06–2007/08*. London: Department of Health.

Doyal, L., Hunt, G. and Mellow, J. (1980) *Your Life in Their Hands: Migrant Workers in the NHS*. Polytechnic of North London, Department of Sociology – for the Social Science Research Council.

Ehrenreich, B. and English, D. (1979) *For Her Own Good: 100 Years of Advice to Women*. London: Pluto Press.

Evans, J. (1996) *Feminist Theory Today: An Introduction to Second-Wave Feminism*. London: Sage.

Evans, J. (2004) Men nurses: a historical and feminist perspective. *Journal of Advanced Nursing* 47(3): 321–328.

Franklin, B. (2014) *The Future Care Workforce*. Anchor, ILC-UK, www.ilcuk.org.uk.

Freidson, E. (1970) *The Profession of Medicine: A Study of the Sociology of Applied Knowledge*. New York: Dodd, Mead and Co.

Gamarnikov, E. (1978) Sexual division of labour: the case of nursing. In A. Kuhn and A. Wolpe (eds) *Feminism and Materialism*. London: Routledge & Kegan Paul

Gamble, A. (1988) *The Free Economy and the Strong State: The Politics of Thatcherism*. Basingstoke: Macmillan.

Gardell, B., Gustafsson, R., Brandt, C., Tillström, I. and Torbörn, I. (1979) Sjukvård på löpandeband. [Health Care on a Conveyor Belt]. Stockholm: Prismas bokförlöag

Goffman, E. (1956) *The Presentation of Self in Everyday Life*. Monograph No. 2. Edinburgh: University of Edinburgh, Social Sciences Research Centre.

Hardill, I. and Macdonald, S. (2000) Skilled international migration: the experience of nurses in the UK. *Regional Studies* 34(7): 681–692.

Harding, S. (1987) Introduction: is there a feminist method? In S. Harding (ed.) *Feminism and Methodology*. Milton Keynes: Open University Press, pp. 1–14.

Hochschild, A.R. (2003) *The Commercialisation of Intimate Life*. Berkeley, CA: University of California Press.

Holden, T. (2005) *Queen Coal: Women of the Miners' Strike*. Stroud: Sutton Publishing.

Iredale, R. (2001) The migration of professionals: theories and typologies. *International Migration* 39(5): 7–26.

Leonardo, M. di (1991) Introduction: gender, culture and political economy. In M. di Leonardo (ed.) *Gender at the Crossroads of Knowledge*. Berkeley, CA: University of California Press, pp. 1–48.

Letherby, G. (2003) *Feminist Research in Theory and Practice*. Maidenhead: McGraw Hill Education.

Lombard, D. (2012) Why don't men want to work in social care? *Social Care Worker*, 24 October. Available at: www.socialcareworker.co/2012/10/24/why-dontmen-want-to-work-in-social-care/ (accessed 2 September 2015).

Low Pay Commission (2013) *National Minimum Wage*. London: The Stationery Office.

Lowes, R. (2010) Largest ever nurses' strike could be sign of future unrest. *Medscape Medical News*. Available at: www.medscape.com/viewarticle/723437 (accessed 2 September 2015).

Martin, P.Y. (2006) Practising gender at work: further thoughts on reflexivity. *Gender, Work & Organisation* 13(3): 254–276.

Merton, R.K. (1948/1968) *Social Theory and Social Structure*. New York: The Free Press.

Miles, R. (1988) *The Women's History of the World*. London: Paladin Books.

Nelson, S. (2010) The nightingale imperative. In S. Nelson and A.-M. Rafferty (eds) *Notes on Nightingale*. Ithaca, NY: Cornell University Press, pp. 9–27.

Nursing and Midwifery Council (NMC) (2005) *Statistical Analysis of the Register: 1 April 2004 to 31 March 2005*. London: Nursing and Midwifery Council.

Nursing and Midwifery Council (NMC) (2011) *Statistical Analysis of the Register: 1 April 2010–31 March 2011*. London: Nursing and Midwifery Council.

Oakley, A. (1974) *The Sociology of Housework*. Oxford: Basil Blackwell.

Oakley, A. (1986) On the importance of being a nurse. In *Telling the Truth about the New Jerusalem: A Collection of Essays and Poems*. Oxford: Basil Blackwell, pp. 180–195.

Pearson, M. (1985) *Equal Opportunities in the NHS: A Handbook*. Cambridge: National Extension College for Training in Race and Health.

Platzer, H. (1988) Redressing the balance. *Nursing Standard* 2(15): 42.

Porter, S. (1992) Women in a women's job: the gendered experiences of nurses. *Sociology of Health & Illness* 14: 510–517.

Proctor, S. (2000) *Caring for Health*. London: Macmillan.

Rankin, J.M. and Campbell, M. (2009) Institutional Ethnography (IE), nursing work and hospital reform: IE's cautionary analysis. *Forum: Qualitative Social Research* 10(2): Art. 8. Available at: www.qualitative-research.net/ (accessed 21 September 2014).

Robertson, M.M. (1992) Lesbians as an invisible minority in the health services arena. *Health Care for Women International* 13(2): 155–163.

Rose, P. (1993) Out in the open? *Lesbianism. Nursing Times* 89: 30, 50–5.

Salvage, J. (1985) *The Politics of Nursing*. London: Heinemann.

Seccombe, I. and Ball, J. (1992) *Motivation, Morale and Mobility: a Profile of Qualified Nurses in the 1990s*. London: Institute of Manpower Studies.

Simpson, R. (2011) Men discussing women and women discussing men: reflexivity, transformation and gendered practice in the context of nursing care. *Gender, Work & Organisation* 18(4): 377–398.

Skills for Care (2013) *The Size and Structure of the Adult Social Care Sector and Workforce in England, 2013*. Available at: www.skillsforcare.org.uk/Documentlibrary/NMDS-SC-Workforce-intelligence-publications/The-size-and-structure-of-the-adult-social-care-sector-and-workforce-in-England.aspx (accessed 7 January 2016).

Siddique, H. (2015) New immigration rules will cost the NHS millions, warns nursing union, *Guardian*, 22 June. Available at: www.theguardian.com/society/2015/jun/22/new-immigration-rules-cost-nhs-millions-nursing (accessed 1 September 2015).

Smith, P. (1987) Mary Seacole. In M. McNeil (ed.) *Gender and Expertise*. London, Free Association Books.

Smith, P. (1992) *The Emotional Labour of Nursing: How Nurses Care*. Basingstoke: Palgrave Macmillan.

Smith, P. (2012) *The Emotional Labour of Nursing Revisited: Can Nurses Still Care?* 2nd edition. Basingstoke: Palgrave Macmillan.

Smith, P., Allan, H., Henry, L., Larsen, J. and Mackintosh, M (2006) *Valuing and Recognising the Talents of a Diverse Healthcare Workforce. January 2004–June 2006*. Available at: www.rcn.org.uk/professional-development/publications/pub-003078.

Smith, P. and Mackintosh, M. (2007) Profession market and class: nurse migration and the re-making of division and disadvantage. *Journal of Clinical Nursing* 16(12): 2213–2220.

Smith, P., Mackintosh, M. and Towers, B. (1993) Implications of the new NHS contracting system for the District Nursing Service in One Health Authority. *Journal of Interprofessional Care* 7(2): 115–124.

Stalker, P. (2000) *Workers without Frontiers: The Impact of Globalization on International Migration*. Boulder, CO: Lynne Rienner Publishers.

Stanley, L. and Wise, S. (1993) *Breaking Out Again: Feminist Ontology and Epistemology*. New edition. London: Routledge.

Street, A.F. (1992) *Inside Nursing: A Critical Ethnography of Clinical Nursing Practice*. New York: State University of New York.

UK Government (2010) *Equality Act*. London: UK Government.

Towers, B. Smith, P. and Mackintosh, M. (1999) Dimensions of class in the integration of health and social care. *Journal of Interprofessional Care* 13(3): 219–228.

Traynor, M. (1999) *Managerialism and Nursing: Beyond Profession and Oppression*. London: Routledge.

Ungerson, C. (1983) Women and caring: skills, tasks and taboos. In E. Gamarnikov, D. Morgan, J. Purvis and D. Taylorson (eds) *The Public and the Private*. London: Heinemann.

Ungerson, C. (2006) Care, work and feeling. *The Sociological Review* 53(2): 188–203.

Villeneuve, M. (1994) Recruiting and retaining men in nursing: a review of the literature. *Journal of Professional Nursing* 10(4): 217–228.

Vinen, R. (2009) *Thatcher's Britain: The Politics and Social Upheaval of the 1980s*. London: Simon & Schuster

Walby, S. (1987) *Gender Politics*, Working paper.

Walby, S. (1990) *Theorising Patriarchy*. Oxford: Basil Blackwell.

Warwick-Booth, L. (2013) *Social Inequality*. London: Sage.

Whittock, M., Edwards, C., McLaren, S. and Robinson, O. (2002) The tender trap: gender, part-time nursing and the effects of 'family friendly' policies on career advancement. *Sociology of Health and Illness* 24(3): 305–326.

Wilkinson, G. and Miers, M. (1999) *Power and Nursing Practice*. Basingstoke: Macmillan.

Witz, A. (1990) *Professions and Patriarchy*. London: Routledge.

5

Caring, face-work and nursing

Daniel Kelly and Pam Smith

The issue

The issue or concern in this chapter is the emotional nature of nursing work; we emphasise that caring is an emotional as well as a physical activity. Each interaction with a patient elicits an emotional reaction and sometimes these emotions can present challenges for nurses. Emotional reactions are sometimes difficult to contain and manage yet the professional code that nurses are bound by, the Nursing & Midwifery Council (NMC) Code, clearly states our duty is to care for everyone in a dignified way. In this chapter we will explore some sociological concepts about caring work as well as the question of how the presentation of caring as 'face-work' can be understood from a sociological perspective. We will also invite you to think about emotional labour and the need to be aware of the stress you may experience as a nurse, and, by being aware of expectations placed upon you, to care for yourself as well as others.

Consider the following:

You put the interests of people using or needing nursing or midwifery services first. You make their care and safety your main concern and make sure that their dignity is preserved and their needs are recognised, assessed and responded to. You make sure that those receiving care are treated with respect, that their rights are upheld and that any discriminatory attitudes and behaviours towards those receiving care are challenged.

The fundamentals of care include, but are not limited to, nutrition, hydration, bladder and bowel care, physical handling and making sure that those receiving care are kept in clean and hygienic conditions. It includes making sure that those receiving care have adequate access to nutrition and hydration, and making sure that you provide help to those who are not able to feed themselves or drink fluid unaided. (NMC Code, published January 2015, effective from March 2015)

Consider these questions:

- Is it always possible to put your patients first, and to treat them with respect and in a dignified way?
- Are the fundamentals of care always delivered respectfully and in a dignified way in your placements and if not, why not?
- Do nurses no longer care? If so, why do they not care?

Now consider the following extract from Pam Smith's article entitled 'Counter the scapegoating and show the public you still care' in *Nursing Times*, February 2013:

Hardly a day goes by without nurses being put in the line of fire for their lack of care and compassion. Robert Francis' report of the Mid Staffordshire Foundation Trust inquiry inevitably intensified the focus. The quality of nursing care came under intense scrutiny where, for a variety of reasons, nurses appeared to be unable to provide care that met patients' physical and emotional needs. Staff, relatives and patients lived in an atmosphere where they were afraid to speak out about failures in care.

The profession needs to brace itself to address and go beyond the Francis report and counter the scapegoating of nursing by drawing on the wisdom and experience of generations of nurses to show once again to the public how nurses still care.

In this chapter we will offer you a sociological view of emotions in nursing, by which we mean we look at emotions arising from the interactions between patients, their families and carers but they are set within the context of the social structures and systems in which they take place. This is in keeping with our approach to nursing through a consideration of micro (in this case, emotions) and macro sociology (the setting or context in which the emotions arise).

Chapter outline

In this chapter we will introduce you to the following:

- Why nurses are expected to care
  - The concept of face-work and emotional authenticity
  - Emotional labour and nursing work
  - Emotions and the everyday work of nurses
- The commodification of care
  - The link between caring, compassion and the culture of healthcare
- The idea of the 'new model nurse'
- Being aware of the emotional demands of caring work, shifts and the need to balance the stress of nursing with your own well-being.

Introduction

In this chapter we focus on the emotional aspects of nursing as work and the challenges that you may face when dealing with illness, suffering, pain and death. This is not easy, especially when other people would never be expected to engage with such situations in their working lives, and so we invite you to think about the types of roles that nurses are expected to adopt, and the events you will become involved in, from a sociological perspective. Key to this chapter is the relationship between what you will be expected to *do* as a nurse and the *attitudes* expected of you (from your patients, other colleagues or your lecturers) as you do it. Your work is also being regulated by the NMC and the Code that is intended to govern the standards that nurses adopt – extracts from this Code were used to open this chapter and you will notice that the tone is one of expectation and emphasises the expectation that nurses will respond to the vulnerability of patients. In Chapter 7 we will explore further the issues of care standards, especially in relation to scandals and the lessons that may be drawn.

We will also encourage you to consider whether institutions (such as the National Health Service – NHS) are organised to help you to respond in a way that demonstrates authentic caring, or whether the context of your nursing practice may make this goal very challenging.

Using a sociological perspective we invite you to think about the unique expectation placed on nurses to demonstrate 'caring attitudes' towards strangers during their working day. We will draw on the concepts of 'dramaturgy' and 'emotional labour' to help you think about how we might present ourselves as caring, but also the extent to which this can always be authentic. This will need you to adopt a more objective stance on why caring might be an important attitude or skill in practice, but it is also a valuable resource when people expect caring attitudes from nurses. We then invite you to consider the value placed on caring by society. To work as a nurse, however, you should also be aware of your own emotional limits and resilience. Throughout this book we invite you to link theory with your own practice experiences. Using the sociological perspective we can help you, as the French sociologist Pierre Bourdieu suggested, to 'reveal that which is hidden'.

Why are nurses expected to care?

This is an important question that could be asked to anyone involved in healthcare (including doctors, other members of the team or NHS managers). However, it is to nurses that society looks when seeking a caring response in healthcare services. This suggests that the nursing role is connected strongly with an expectation to care. When we think of roles we can understand them in different ways. One way is to think of everyday life as a form of theatre in which we adopt different roles for different situations. Thus we can become a *character*, with an expectation to *act* in certain ways and to *say* certain *lines*, in the right *order* and on *cue*.

The theatrical comparison is a central component of the theory of dramaturgy. This is one of the central pillars of the American sociologist Erving Goffman's work, including his book *The Presentation of Self in Everyday Life*. This was first published in the late 1950s and has been listed as one of the ten most important sociology books of the twentieth century.

The central argument within this chapter is that when we come into contact with other people we try to manage the impression they have of us, by presenting a certain 'face', so we may present one face to our friends, another to our parents and another to the patients we meet on a hospital ward. Goffman argues that one of the main drivers of the 'face-work' that we engage in is to avoid social embarrassment. So we learn to act appropriately in the 'front stage' arena (by the patient's bed we may act as if we care about them) but in another way when we interact in the 'backstage' with our colleagues (where we may try to come across as confident and unaffected by what we are doing).

There is a simple example of Goffman's theory of embarrassment avoidance in action. Once when he went out for dinner with friends he ordered a dessert when everyone else ordered starters. This threw the waiter into a state of confusion and embarrassed the accompanying guests. Goffman was able to demonstrate the importance of the 'social script', and the rules that governed the 'front stage' actions in a restaurant setting. Think about how you or patients have to cope with social rules and potential embarrassment – by getting things wrong or being unable to do things (such as wash) that we would normally do unheeded in a private backstage setting.

However, it is sometimes difficult to maintain the different faces that we try to adopt as student nurses, as the following example from Pam's study of how students learn to care shows.

Scenario 5.1

A third-year student tells me about an incident in which she was involved in caring for an unconscious patient whose condition suddenly deteriorates. She calls the ward sister, who comes quickly to the patient's bedside followed closely by two doctors. The student is told immediately to suction the secretions from the patient's airway. The sister's tone is cold and mechanical. The student quickly dons gloves, assembles the suction equipment and turns on the suction machine. She then moves purposefully towards the patient and begins to insert the suction catheter into his mouth to take away any secretions which may have caused him to choke. In her haste to obey the sister's instructions, she forgets the golden rule 'before any procedure always tell the patient, even when unconscious, what you are going to do'. Her omission immediately provokes the sister to snap at her for failing to warn the patient that he was about to be subject to an invasive procedure.

The student is so shocked and upset at being spoken to in this way that before she knows what is happening there are tears streaming down her cheeks. She swallows hard to conceal any sounds and hopes that the sister will not notice as she recovers herself sufficiently to carry on with the suctioning procedure. The sister and doctors nudge each other and exchange meaningful glances about the student's tears, but do not say anything to her, either in comfort or as a reprimand. She leaves the patient's bedside at the

first possible opportunity and goes straight to the bathroom where she immediately bursts into the sobs she has suppressed in public.

Later, she told me the reasons for her reactions. First, she had felt tense and
anxious at the patient's sudden deterioration. Second, suctioning patients to
clear their airway was still a relatively unfamiliar and frightening procedure to
her, so that she had been concentrating hard on the technical task in hand.

When the sister abruptly broke into her concentration, she was genuinely
startled, then shocked and humiliated that she had overlooked such a basic
principle as to warn the patient of the impending procedure. She felt even
more humiliated when the sister and doctors, rather than being sympathetic,
reacted in a humiliating way. She felt that the sister had made her look stupid
in front of the doctors and had undermined her confidence. (Smith, 1992: 72)

In this account we can see the face-work theory at first hand. The student nurse is
obviously very aware of the need to adopt a competent and caring role (informing
others of the patient's deterioration) but she is then embarrassed and loses face in
front of more experienced colleagues (trying to hide her feelings of upset).

Note also the face-work and role adopted by the ward sister who speaks in an
unsupportive way to the student and seems instead to locate her allegiance with the
doctors rather than the student. This may be a way of her maintaining her own
sense of competence and avoiding the embarrassment caused by the student's emotional reactions. Everyone in the situation can be seen to have adopted a role and
followed a non-emotional script; the student was not following the same script and
the outcome was a student who felt humiliated whilst everyone else was left intact
as competent 'social actors'.

Reflection 5.1

When you read this incident how does it make you feel? Do you think there is
anything positive for the student nurse to take away from this event? If you
have ever felt unsure of the role you are expected to adopt (maybe when you
go to a new placement) how did you manage this feeling? What have you
learned about face-work and being a nursing student?

Face-work and emotional authenticity

Understanding the importance of face-work allows us to question the link between
recognition of emotions in our work and why they are important in the context of
how we demonstrate caring in nursing. There are different ways of understanding
this. One position is:

Emotions are pivotal to understanding, both about ourselves and the caring relationships made in the social world with others, so have particular relevance for health and social carers who are required to engage with the feelings of patients and families as a matter of routine. (Gray, 2012: 1)

Alternatively, another researcher suggests if we do not focus more attention on the importance of emotions in our work then, 'Much of nurses' work remains unnoticed or uncounted' (Ruchti, 2012: 54).

Reflection 5.2

Take a few minutes to consider Gray and Ruchti's statements and jot down a few of your own thoughts on the importance of emotions at work as a nurse.

Pam's study (Smith, 1992) referred to above was undertaken in the 1980s when many student nurses were apprentices and part of the workforce. One of the main discoveries was that it was the work of the ward sister or charge nurse that was so important in supporting the students to care by setting the emotional tone, which, in turn, created a 'caring climate'. Students recognised the caring climate as a good place to learn. As one student commented during an interview: 'You can only learn to care in a caring climate.' When the student was asked to comment further on what she meant by a 'caring climate', she said: 'When I know that the ward sister [charge nurse] cares then I feel a bit more at ease. Otherwise I feel that I have to take the whole caring attitude of the whole ward on my shoulders.' Another student added: 'Sisters [charge nurses] are critical because of their influence on staff nurses. They in turn influence how the students work and on the way they feel, their morale.' Yet another student described how negative as well as positive emotions had an effect on learning and caring: 'Fear isn't a good way to learn to care. Mutual respect is the best. If you feel appreciated you try to live up to the faith people have in you. It's a very strong stimulus.'

The 'caring climate' also meant recognising and valuing the 'little things' or 'gestures of caring' (an extension of face-work perhaps?) such as holding the hand of an anxious patient, or making sure the older patient's hearing aid work or wrapping the shivering patient in a blanket to keep them warm. However, these 'little things' or 'gestures of caring' are difficult to capture and may slip by unnoticed in the daily routines and hustle and bustle of ward life. The earlier point about noticing the roles that people adopt in work situations may help to make clear when caring gestures are authentic or not. Doing something because 'it is the done thing' may not be quite the same as doing something because you feel the need to step outside of what is usually expected of you and demonstrate care for a patient. The examples above, however, emphasise that the face-work we engage in as nurses is sometimes scripted and often 'directed' by the person in charge of the ward or unit. Learning to see their behaviour as a role (with a script) can help to understand why they act as they do – and may also offer alternative ways to act ourselves.

Reflection 5.3

Can you think of some of the 'little things' that you may have observed or been involved with that have made a difference to a patient, a relative, a fellow student or member of staff? Was this an everyday behaviour or did it require a change to make this caring act occur?

When Pam asked student nurses in a more recent study into student nurse learning (O'Driscoll et al., 2010) if they could recall any of the 'little things' or 'caring gestures' that had made a difference, this was one response given: '[care] … it's a lot of the little things and I definitely like chatting to patients and asking them if they're alright, if they slept okay, have they got any worries?' (Smith, 2012: 2).

Helen, one of the co-authors of this book, was also involved in this later study to find out who was and what was influential in shaping the learning and caring that took place in hospital wards (Allan et al., 2008; Smith, 2012).

The study found that sisters/charge nurses' roles had changed over recent years and their work now included increased management responsibilities, which distanced them from direct contact with patients, nurses and students. The clinical mentor had taken on the role of caring for both students and patients and supporting their learning about how to adopt the role of competent nurse. One mentor in the study mentioned how the 'little things' made a difference to students: 'I think the students value just being made welcome and little things like being shown where the off duty is and where they can put their coat and it's the friendly side of it, yeah. They do appreciate that' (Smith, 2012: 2). This is a simple gesture but is an example of the mentor choosing to adopt a 'caring script' that humanises the student and makes them feel welcome as an individual in this setting. Once again there is authenticity in the interaction that is passed to the student nurse – it is simple but it is powerful. With patients the corollary is the little things mentioned above – they are simple yet powerful symbols of individuality and caring attitudes.

In this research, as in the earlier study 25 years previously, it was found that when students felt cared for themselves they were better able to care for patients. They gave many examples of the friendliness shown towards them, the building up of good relationships and their confidence to care. One student described in detail one mentor who stood out for her 'right from the start' who

completely listened to everything that I wanted to do, suggested things that would be beneficial to me and took the time out, if I didn't understand something, to actually sit down with me and go through it, and she actually arranged when we were working nights and it wasn't particularly busy on that ward, she actually spent the time to do some teaching sessions with me. Another thing I think is that they've made me feel like it's a safe environment to actually have a go and build my confidence up in doing that. I think encouragement as well. (Smith, 2012: 124)

So being aware of the role your mentors can play can help you to build your confidence, which, in turn, can help you to learn about good patient care and how to put this into practice. Mentors can help you learn the 'script' of being a competent and caring nurse, but this must be matched with technical competence and confidence. This takes time and you must not expect to master the skills necessary in a short time. The comment from the student in the first study that 'fear is not a good way to learn' but mutual respect and appreciation is best still holds true today and will be important to remember as you become mentors to students in the future.

'Seeing both sides'

Another point to emphasise is that some students had learned to see the practice situations they found themselves in from both sides. This meant that they could understand why attention could not always be paid to them due to heavy workload. In Goffman's terms they had learned to appreciate other people's roles and the limitations of caring 'scripts'.

One student gave an example:

> I can think of when I was in ICU on my very first day and my mentor was looking after two patients and one of the patients just went really downhill and his focus was not me as a student but was on the patient, which ultimately is what it should be. And at the end of it he said to me 'I'm so sorry I've not been able to show you this and this' and I'm like 'look, it doesn't matter, we've got plenty of time and that priority was the patient and not me', and I think as students you've sometimes got to be aware of that as well. (From original interview transcript for Allan et al., 2008).

Another student who had the ward manager as her mentor noted:

> Because I was a third year and nearing the end of my training, and because obviously the ward manager has got so much to do I think it helped her when she was on the ward because obviously I was working with her, so I took some of her workload off her. (Smith, 2012: 120)

Another aspect of seeing both sides for some students was being aware not only that mentors might also have needs but that caring should revolve around the patients rather than students. A third-year student said:

> Some students think that the ward revolves around them don't they? But it doesn't, it revolves around the patients and ... you have to go out there and get what you want from the placement. But you know it's about being flexible. (Smith, 2012: 121)

Her colleague responded: 'Yeah ... it is swings and roundabouts you know, you get what you put in' (Smith, 2012: 121).

So caring is not just about having the right 'script' or doing the right 'face-work' but is about authenticity, empathy with others and 'seeing both sides'. Thus as an empathic student nurse you will be learning many things at once – not least the skill of recognising other people's needs in a given situation and responding in a way that promotes a caring environment based on the development of rapport, effective communication and respectful working relationships.

You may think that this is all very well – especially the point made by one of the students that caring should always revolve round the patients. However, you will also expect some support to stay authentic and you may now wish to refer to Chapters 4 and 8 to read about how organisations and hierarchy can constrain the way work is organised and delegated. Chapter 7 also explores when things go wrong and when face-work and scripts combine to create workplace cultures that are abnormally negative, and sometimes destructive in character.

Reflection 5.4

How does a good mentor make you feel? What are the effects on your learning and caring when you feel welcomed to the team? Does this impact on how you approach learning to fit and learn the script of each setting? Do you feel that your attitude is more authentic towards the patients?

In the next section we introduce the concept of emotional labour, which builds further on Goffman's theory of face-work as well as how we act in 'front-stage' and 'backstage' spaces at work. We then introduce further influential sociologically relevant research by Isabel Menzies that provides a provocative insight into the way that nurses and healthcare professionals deal with the stresses of their work. The way they rely on the scripts (and turn them into tasks and routines) may limit their ability to connect with individual patients. This type of care may be technically competent but emotionally limited. We will end by thinking about how you might build up your own resilience to become someone who can enjoy your work as a nurse and gain a sense of achievement from it.

Emotional labour and nursing work

The concept of emotional labour was first developed by another American sociologist, Arlie Hochschild, in the 1980s. She observed flight attendants employed on Delta Airlines and observed the nature of their work closely by focusing on the attitudes they were expected to adopt and the emotional displays required of them in their work. She described the way they were expected to smile and present a positive and friendly attitude and to make the paying passengers feel safe and 'cared for'. She termed this kind of work 'emotional labour' and it has come to be used to explore the demands placed on nursing and the way that expectations to work at an emotionally appropriate manner may be constrained by the systems through which healthcare is delivered.

Since Hochschild's work was published there has been a range of research into this topic, including the work described above by Smith (1992, 2012) in nursing, and by Hunter (2004) in midwifery.

We would encourage you to think about emotional labour not only as a theoretical issue but also in relation to your own emotional experiences as a student nurse. We also invite you to think how this awareness of working at an emotional level might relate to your capacity to care for patients and families you will meet, and to question – some sociologists would encourage you to 'problematise' – the role that you will eventually be taking on as a registered nurse. There is an obvious link with the face-work and the scripts approach that we have already discussed. These socio-logical concepts help to describe the nature of the work that nurses engage in – and can help us understand the challenges involved in doing so.

However, it is also important to question the social nature of caring because, as we discussed in Chapter 4, it is also linked with the historical roots of nursing and the caring role of women in the domestic arena. Proctor (2000) provides a useful sum-mary of the debates around caring and takes the stance that, because it is so gendered, society fails to recognise the worth of nursing in improving health services on many different levels. Although the argument is not new, she makes the following case that raises some challenging issues in today's context: 'Today, the health service is flounder-ing because it is able to recognize neither the inequality that gender blindness has created for the workforce of the NHS, nor the centrality of the work undertaken by nurses …' (Proctor, 2000: 3). If all aspects of nursing are to be better understood then awareness of emotional labour can also encourage you to think about how you must learn to be aware of your own, or other people's emotions, and how they are managed at the individual level within a clinical situation (such as how you might learn to deal with an angry patient who has been kept waiting for a long time, or a bereaved family who have just lost a relative). We also encourage you to consider emotional labour as a means of thinking about how emotions are changed and shaped by working within large organisations such as hospitals. By considering the front-stage features of emo-tional labour, you may also recognise that, as an individual, you need to unwind and recharge in the backstage arena in order to cope. Backstage in this context can mean backstage in the clinical setting by having informal conversations or sharing jokes, or relaxing at home with family or friends. Awareness of your own engagement in emo-tional labour may, in turn, impact on how aware you are of feeling stressed in practice, such as when there is not enough time to deal with a patient's needs.

We hope you will use the insights in this chapter to evaluate the expectations that exist around the emotional aspects of the care you will be expected to provide as a student nurse by thinking about emotional labour and its relevance to your devel-oping skills. As a registered nurse you will be expected to 'care' by your patients, your employers and by society more generally. This might be expected to include having a 'caring' demeanour when you are carrying out your work. Whilst this is something you may have thought about already, we hope you will see the expecta-tion to display your caring emotions as an issue worth further analysis.

Reflection 5.5

To do this we encourage you to reflect on the role of emotions in your learning and clinical experiences. Think about how it feels to 'give' to other people on a daily basis and the ways that this makes you feel. Do you feel rewarded by it? Do you find it tiring? Is it dependent primarily on the situation (who the person in charge is, perhaps, as we suggested earlier?) and how motivated you feel?

These are not complex sociological issues but they are key to understanding the importance of the setting and teams in which you are working. Each setting will feel different as you proceed through your training, each will have their own routines, and it is helpful to develop an awareness of this and question the *culture* of the workplace you are in.

As you move through this chapter we emphasise that care is an emotional, as well as a physical, process and is a complex and challenging issue in modern-day nursing.

Emotions and the everyday work of nurses

In this section we introduce you to the work of Isabel Menzies, a psychoanalyst who carried out influential research in the late 1950s in English hospitals (Menzies, 1960). Her conclusions have been considered fairly radical ever since as she suggested that student nurses who did not complete their training tended to be those who were more 'mature and thoughtful' in their outlook. She also suggested that those who stayed were the ones who could take orders and 'fit in' to the routines that shaped the nature of hospital life (think here of the link with Goffman's scripts and the social importance of 'fitting in').

She emphasised particularly the role that routines played in protecting nurses from what she called 'anxiety' – a rather general term for a feeling of emotional discomfort – which implied the negative feelings that might be experienced by engaging with patients' emotional needs and their suffering. Here we can see the emergence of stress as an outcome of engaging with patients as individuals.

As we suggested earlier in this chapter when thinking about the concept of emotional labour, the contribution of Isabel Menzies' research adds to our understanding of the subtle social forces that come into play during the everyday work of being a nurse.

Reflection 5.6

Think about a typical day on a busy surgical ward. As a relatively new student nurse you are keen to fit in and to learn as much as you can. At the morning handover you are asked to work with an experienced staff nurse who is also known as a good teacher, but expects high standards of care. As you are given a group of patients she tells you about the pre-operative care that will be needed for those going to theatre that day – you will also be caring for two post-operative patients. One of these patients has cancer of the liver and is awaiting important biopsy results.

As you think about the day ahead can you consider the emotions that patients and families may be experiencing? How do these emotions of the patients make you feel? How do you think you might you respond? Does it feel easier if you have a list of things to do and you can feel busy and useful?

(Continued)

(Continued)

Does knowing the routine help you? How does it feel when there is not so much to do? How might you feel about engaging in conversations with patients awaiting important results?

What might you learn from observing how the experienced nurse deals with the patients and their families?

Now think about whether you have had experience of clinical situations where you felt more engaged in the emotional aspects of care? Think about such a situation now and how this made you feel? Have you witnessed more experienced nurses dealing well with patients who were worried? How did they do this and how did the patients react? Try to think about situations where this seemed to go well, and some others where it did not.

Can you now think about the skills, resources and support you might need to carry out 'emotional labour' well?

We hope you will agree by now that all healthcare settings are emotional as well as physical spaces. Theodosius (2008: 5) argues that this is the case irrespective of the care they offer. There are many examples in various research studies.

One example is the findings that gynaecology wards have been described as 'women's places' where nurses wanted to give their emotional labour as 'a gift' to the women (Bolton, 2000).

Another example is the prostate cancer ward. Daniel, one of the authors of this book, described how men, normally less likely to share emotions, looked after each other and came to demonstrate what was termed a new kind of masculinity where emotions were evident and caring was more present than in everyday life – albeit that it was highly gendered in nature (Kelly, 2009).

There are also many examples you can probably think of from other contexts, such as emergency mental healthcare, where Hochschild's and Menzies' theories will be seen in action.

A student nurse from Pam's 1980s study that was introduced earlier described the mechanisms used on a psychiatric ward to focus on the emotional aspects of the work. She described what happened when feelings ran high for both patients and staff.

If there was an intense staff interaction, say when the patient's being very aggressive and you get upset. It would be put directly to someone in charge. Everything would stop. There would be a discussion. It wouldn't just be 'what should we do about this?' First of all the trained staff would start on you. 'How does this upset you? Are you sure you feel alright? This plan of action isn't working with this patient. Let's go and talk to them and let them know.' (Smith, 1992: 56–57)

The focus of work on the psychiatric ward was clearly defined around relationships and feelings and how to manage them systematically. The person in charge would stop 'everything' to discuss a patient care issue and how it affected the nurses.

This account illustrates some of the emotional stress and tensions surrounding the emergency care of acutely ill patients. It also demonstrate the effects of the leadership style on the emotional well-being of patients and nurses. Whilst routines might exist on the ward, there was also room to stop and consider that was needed to deal with the situation.

Another example can be found in a PhD that Daniel was involved in supervising (Kelly and Kelly, 2013). This was about the experiences of children of Bangladeshi heritage who were undergoing treatment for cancer. Using an ethnographic approach (observing events as they occur over a prolonged period) it was possible to understand the ways that parents also learned to find ways round the ward routine to provide emotional support to their child. Here is a short extract.

Scenario 5.2

Following the cancer diagnosis parents embarked on a careful balancing act, involving the demonstration of appropriate and prompt degrees of contact with the hospital balanced with recognition that the clinical staff had other children to care for. Parents of children with cancer were at times required to temper their own worries and anxieties, or risk being labelled as a parent who found it 'difficult to cope'. In the hospital context particularly parents were expected to recognise competing demands from other patients:

The child has now been in this ward for five days. It is Sunday evening and she and I are playing a board game. Her mother looks at the clock. 'She was due her antibiotics at 5pm and it's nearly 6pm now. I am going to ask the nurse who is looking after her if she is going to have it at 6pm. They gave it this morning at 5 so I think it should be 5pm tonight, that is right.' She comes back a little while later. 'I found the nurse who is getting it ready,' she says. 'She is in a line, she has 12 to do so she is in the line they will get to her.'

In this example the mother used her knowledge about the appropriateness of treatment times, but balanced this with the context of other demands placed on the ward nurses' time. Her work involved employing vigilance and an advocacy role, superimposed on her own anxieties about the potential effects of delayed treatment within an organisation that she had little power to influence.

Each example given so far in this chapter illustrates the way that routines are features of hospital life, but, with greater awareness of their role and importance, it is possible for health professionals, and patients and families, to challenge or to bend them to derive a more desirable outcome.

However, the social importance of caring behaviours goes beyond clinical interactions. They are also seen as something valuable to both patients and to healthcare organisations who require caring staff in order to function and thrive. Without it, they may be efficient, but soulless, places.

The commodification of care

As well as the personal/attitudinal dimension of care, we can also explore it on a larger, societal scale. At this level the way that nurses act can also be viewed as a social commodity; that is, a limited resource with some value to people or organisations who need it. When applied to healthcare, therefore, the term care can be used in ways that implies that whole organisations can care, rather than the individuals who make up the many departments, units and wards. So we might see the NHS adopting phrases where the value attached to 'good care' for patients is interwoven into statements using a more business-like philosophy.

In the box below you can see how this mix of sentiments was displayed in an anonymous advertisement for a senior nursing role in a fictitious NHS organisation.

Scenario 5.3

Nightingale NHS Trust is a dynamic and exciting place to work. The unique way we deliver services and offer everyone who works here a voice means that your career with us will be rewarding.

Nightingale NHS Trust has three key tenets and we want to employ and work with people who share these values and demonstrate behaviours that support them. They are:

- to constantly improve our services;
- to treat people as we would like to be treated ourselves;
- to hit our targets.

You will notice the use of the phrase 'to treat people as we would like to be treated ourselves'. This is akin to the ideal espoused by many religions as the Golden Rule and emphasises the interpersonal element of most caring philosophies. To present care as a desirable quality in this way illustrates its inherent value to healthcare organisations, such as the fictitious Nightingale Trust above. This also introduces another important sociological concept that can be applied to care – viewing it as a finite resource, or a commodity, that has social (and financial) value.

However, the way that this is achieved is via the actions and attitudes of individual employees that make up large NHS organisations. Therefore, we invite you to think about your attitudes to care for patients as having value on different levels. This might start with individual interactions that help patients feel safe and satisfied that their needs are being met. Then your attitudes to others will have value at the level of the team where you can be trusted to take responsibility and work with others to help make the hospital function. On a larger scale the way that the individual works will shape the reputation of the organisation as a whole in things like patient-satisfaction surveys. So your contribution to the NHS is more than you might think and your caring skills have value. You may want to look at the debate in

Chapter 4 about nursing as work and the way that nursing has fought to obtain pay and working conditions that match the value of care to society as a whole. With fewer nurses, the value attached to their skills will rise, and conversely if their supply increases then their value will fall – a classic supply and demand theory espoused by Karl Marx as long ago as 1844 (see Chapter 1).

> If the supply greatly exceeds the demand, then one section of the workers sinks into beggary or starvation. The existence of the worker is, therefore, reduced to the same condition as the existence of every other commodity. The worker has become a commodity, and he is lucky if he can find a buyer. And the demand on which the worker's life depends is regulated by the whims of the wealthy and the capitalists. (Marx, 1844: 1)

By thinking of the inherent value of your caring skills you might have a better understanding of their (and your) value to society. On a personal level you can choose to work where you prefer, or for an employer who pays more. With advanced skills and competence you can exert even more control over how you use the value of the skills you have. This presents a different way of seeing nursing as a profession with potential in a market where caring skills are needed more and more (just think of the rising numbers of older people who will require the care of nurses in the future). The present, however, as we saw in Chapter 4, is always shaped by history and it is worth another quick look at why nursing has become so closely associated with the provision of care for those who require it in society.

The new model nurse?

The expectation that nurses will care is an interesting and complex topic from a sociological perspective. In historical terms nursing (and healthcare generally) began to be formalised into a profession in the nineteenth century with the 'new model nurse' (Rafferty, 1996). Medicine was also developing from the period of the Enlightenment onwards; however, doctors only became registered under the Medical Registration Act of 1858 (Porter, 2003). Registration for Nursing in the United Kingdom did not come until 1919 and this followed a lengthy process of political and social debate. Hospitals who had always trained nurses preferred to register them as this gave them control over who they employed and their terms and conditions. However, Ethel Bedford-Fenwick championed state registration – something that Florence Nightingale had opposed as she felt the 'moral character' of nurses could not be a subject of teaching or control. This was an interesting point of shift in the expectations that emerged, and still are being placed on nursing today by those who criticise nursing as a graduate-entry profession.

On the one hand there was a drive towards registration (and an associated degree of social status and even professionalisation), and on the other there was the opposite situation where nursing was being presented as a moral cause that relied on the character of the new model nurse. The source of the latter position reflected the historical roots of nursing in religious and service roles.

As time passed we have arrived at a situation where nursing remains a somewhat conflicted occupation. On the one hand nurses may strive to be seen as professionals with university-level education whilst they also come under criticism for being 'uncaring', 'too clever to care' or 'too posh to wash'.

This state of conflict continues and is exemplified in relation to the topic of care and what expectations are placed on nurses by society – such as the levels of engagement that you may need to display so that a patient will feel they are being 'cared for'.

In other words we all have expectations about some social situations – such as how we would wish to be treated if we go into hospital – and we may well feel disappointed if our expectations are not met. A patient in the Nightingale Trust might expect to be feel very well cared for (as the Trust had promised so publicly in the statement above) but may actually be left feeling unhappy if the nurses or doctors, for whatever reason, failed to meet their expectations.

In this situation we begin to see that care is not only a way of relating to each other, as two of the authors we considered in this chapter – Hochschild and Menzies – described it, but it is also a *social commodity*. By this we have suggested that care is something that has some value to society and could be expected to have monetary value and associated social importance. The question remains whether its value is appreciated – except when it is obviously lacking (see Chapter 7).

Authentic caring vs cynicism?

When you are engaged in an activity (in this case caring for others) and you are being paid for it then the source of motivation is not the same as if the person involved is someone you love. Thus we can start to distinguish between *professional* and *lay* caring (Kelly, 1998). We may be highly motivated to care for family or significant others because of their relationship to us; however, in our working lives as nurses we are expected to care for patients, often at increasingly high rates and with the appropriate caring face/attitude. This is an interesting position from a sociological perspective and can lead to questions about what motivates us (beyond our salary) and what happens when we feel less inclined to carry on working where we do. This can have an impact on our inclination to care about others, and the work we do (in the case of nursing this means the way we care about our patients or colleagues). This also links with the face-work that we are willing to engage in, as we discussed earlier. If we are presenting a caring face but, in reality, are feeling highly negative then this state of dissonance will inevitably impact on the attitudes we have about our work. We will now explore briefly the reasons why nurses may feel less engaged in the workplace as this will impact on their ability to care.

Recent research provides two examples that we can draw on to explore this question further. The first concerns those nurses who may feel cynicism towards their work. This is a significant issue as nursing has been found to be one of the occupations that display the highest levels of cynicism (Leiter et al., 2010). By this we mean nurses can feel frustrated, pessimistic, distrustful or even contemptuous towards their job and employers (Wanous et al., 2000). There are various reasons why this may be so. Some researchers have suggested that this can include excessive and unrelenting job demands, lack of resources and low levels of trust in managers (Kim et al., 2009). This is important as nurses may stay in jobs that they dislike for a long time due to a number of reasons, such as family circumstances, avoiding loss of seniority or being too close to retirement to leave (Maertz and Campion, 2004). Whilst they may choose to stay in their role, and display some of the negative attitudes listed above, others may begin to display an 'intention to leave'. This means they would like to move on but do not, or cannot, and so display increasing levels of cynicism.

Once again the concept of face-work becomes important as the cynical nurse may (or may not) 'pretend to care' but actually become passively withdrawn and fails to engage in the work environment beyond the necessary tasks. There are some possible solutions to this situation, such as offering a job change. This can serve to reduce cynicism, but only if the change is agreed to. Those of you who have an interest in becoming leaders will no doubt have to become involved in managing colleagues who have become cynical and withdrawn from their caring role. To motivate them you will certainly face a challenge, and you will need to try different strategies, but this is a situation that is amenable to some degree of resolution if it is acknowledged and managed appropriately (Mantler et al., 2015).

The second example examines the impact of the length of shifts on nurses' ability to work safely and to cope with the fatigue that the job involves. An example of a recent review that looked at this issue can be found at www.england.nhs.uk/6cs/groups/safe-staffing.

This work shows that 12-hour shifts are becoming more prevalent, and that these long hours have been associated with more adverse events, poorer performance, poorer quality of care or higher risks to patient safety. Each of these issues is measured in different ways and adverse events may include, for example, drug errors or 'care left undone' (Ball et al., 2013). What is less easy to measure is the impact on the caring attitudes and motivation of nurses.

Research shows nurses develop different approaches to emotional labour in order to distance themselves from engagement with patients and families such as 'adopting a working persona' (Mackintosh, 2006) and 'self-preservation' strategies (Stayt, 2009). The consequences of working in high-stress environments for prolonged periods have been described as 'burnout' (Maslach and Jackson, 1982). Symptoms include feeling exhausted, detached and emphasising physical over emotional tasks.

Goffman's concept of face-work can again be applied here, and its usefulness comes from understanding the pressures on nurses to maintain a caring attitude when they also may be feeling exhausted and stressed. Alongside this we can return to the work of Isabel Menzies and the importance of routines in protecting nurses from the anxiety induced by dealing with illness and suffering.

Reflection 5.7

You may want to think about the many routines that you may encounter during the 12 hours that a nurse may work on a hospital ward, and how difficult this is to exert any control over when there are multiple demands on your time. You may also want to consider the combination of the culture of the workplace, the way shift rotas are organised, and the emotional and physical aspects of your work and how these impact on the extent to which you can maintain a caring attitude.

Chapter summary

By bringing this chapter to a close we return to you as, what sociologists call, a social agent with choices. By this we mean you can, with insight, exert some degree of control over the situations you find yourself in and have an awareness of the pressures and stress you will encounter if you do work with a caring attitude, and in an authentic way.

The theories presented in this chapter we hope will have helped you to see the social forces at play when we are engaged in the work of nursing. We have introduced you to Goffman's theories of face-work and the relevance of front-stage/backstage contexts. We have also asked you to consider emotional labour as a feature of caring work alongside the power of routines and how they can shape our work in a positive or less positive way. We also talked about care as a commodity with social value and the importance of recognising why some nurses may disengage and become more cynical. Finally, we encourage you think of the routines and shift patterns that will also shape the work you do, and the culture that exists in your workplaces. The other chapters in this book will complement what you have considered here.

Personal resilience and caring

Before we end, however, we want to encourage you to consider your own well-being and to take time to reflect on how you can enjoy your work, and gain personal reward from it.

A piece of recent research that might be helpful in this regard is by Snowden et al. (2014) who explored the relationship between a range of issues such as whether previous caring experience was likely to make nursing students more emotionally intelligent (this is a component of social intelligence and includes the ability to monitor one's own and other people's feelings, to discriminate between them, and to use this to guide one's thinking).

The researchers found that the promotion of mindfulness (developing self-knowledge or well-being through awareness of emotions in the present moment) was more strongly associated with emotional intelligence in student nurses with previous experience in a caring role. Thus you may wish to consider whether a mindful approach to your work – and also your periods of relaxation away from work – might help you in valuing your own well-being as you care for others.

Emotional health is strongly linked with resilience (Rutter, 2012) and we hope you will think about what strategies you could adopt to help you cope with the pressures of nursing. Resilience explores how individuals develop competencies to manage workplace pressures, emotional demands and stress to continue to care for others (McCann et al., 2013). Remember that resilient people also experience negative emotions, but they appear to be able to navigate stress and negative situations with an optimism and positive emotionality (Hunter, 2004; Hart et al., 2014).

By adopting the sociological insights we have offered in this chapter we hope that you will recognise some of the social forces that shape the way you work – and the personal strategies you need to work and thrive both in the 'front-stage' and 'backstage' spaces of your life as a nurse.

Going further

These resources provide additional material that readers may find useful:

Ballatt, J. and Campling, P. (2014) *Intelligent Kindness: Reforming the Culture of Healthcare*. London: Royal College of Psychiatrists.
This book provides a novel way of viewing the NHS as a system with unique value to society, and argues that it needs a new way of looking at how best to promote compassionate practice. Combining both intelligence and kindness is a way to overcome some of the inherent limitations in healthcare policies that fail to ask why staff feel alienated from the system and the patients with whom they work.

Gillett, K. (2014) Nostalgic constructions of nurse education in British national newspapers. *Journal of Advanced Nursing* 70: 2945–2505.
An opportunity to think about the way that the 'model nurse' is constructed – and criticised – by the media. The author provides new insights into the chasm that exists between how the 'face-work' of the caring nurse has become an idealised remnant of the past, rather than acknowledging the complexity of nursing in the present day.

Theodosius, C. (2008) *Emotional Labour in Health Care: The Unmanaged Heart of Nursing*. London: Routledge.
This book takes a different approach to exploring emotional labour and argues that there is need to recognise 'the complex, messy and opaque' nature of emotions that shape the work of nurses and others in healthcare. Since emotion is so strongly linked to communication, its essence can best be understood in relation to identity and the interactions that professionals engage in.

References

Allan, H., Smith, P., Lorentzon. M., O'Driscoll, M. (2008) *Leadership for Learning*. General Nursing Council Trust and the University of Surrey.
Ball, J., Murrells, T., Rafferty, A., Morrow, E. and Griffiths, P. (2013) 'Care left undone' during nursing shifts: associations with workload and perceived quality of care. *BMJ Quality & Safety*. Published online first: DOI 10.1136/BMJQS-2012-001767.
Bolton, S.C. (2000) Who cares? Offering emotion work as a 'gift' in the nursing labour process. *Journal of Advanced Nursing* 32: 580–586.
Bolton, S.C. (2001) Changing faces: nurses as emotional jugglers. *Sociology of Health & Illness* 23: 85–100.
Bolton, S. and Wibberley, G. (2014) Domiciliary care: the formal and informal labour process, *Sociology* 48(4): 682–697.
Goffman, E. (1959) *The Presentation of Self in Everyday Life*. New York: Anchor.
Gray, B. (2012) *Face to Face with Emotions in Health and Social Care*. New York: Springer.
Hart, P.L., Brannan, J.D. and de Chesnay, M. (2014) Resilience in nurses: an integrative review. *Journal of Nursing Management* 22: 720–734.
Hochschild, A. (1983) *The Managed Heart: Commercialisation of Human Feeling*. Berkeley, CA: University of California Press.
Hunter, B. (2004) Conflicting ideologies as a source of emotion work in midwifery. *Midwifery* 20: 261–272.
Kelly, D.M. (1998) Caring and cancer nursing: framing the reality using selected social science theory. *Journal of Advanced Nursing* 28: 728–736.

Kelly, D.M. (2009) Changed men: the embodied impact of prostate cancer. *Qualitative Health Research* 19: 151–163.

Kelly, P. and Kelly, D.M. (2013) Childhood cancer-parenting work for British Bangladeshi families during treatment: an ethnographic study. *International Journal of Nursing Studies* 50: 933–944.

Kim T.-Y., Bateman, T.S., Gilbreath, B. and Andersson, L.M. (2009) Top management credibility and employee cynicism: a comprehensive model. *Human Relations* 62: 1435–1458.

Leiter, M.P., Price, S.L. and Spence Laschinger, H.K. (2010) Generational differences in distress, attitudes, and incivility among nurses. *Journal of Nursing Management* 18: 970–980.

Mackintosh, C. (2006) Protecting the self: a descriptive qualitative exploration of how registered nurses cope with working in surgical areas. *International Journal of Nursing Studies* 44(6): 982–990.

Maertz, C.P. and Campion, M.A. (2004) Profiles in quitting: integrating process and content turnover theory. *Academy of Management* 47: 566–582.

Mantler, J., Godin, J., Cameron, S. and Horsburgh, M. (2015) Cynicism in hospital staff: the effects of intention to leave and job change over time. *Journal of Nursing Management* 23: 577–587.

Marx, K. (1844) *Economic and Philosophical Manuscripts of 1844: Wages of Labour*. Moscow: Prospect Publishers, 1995 Edition. Available at: www.marxists.org/archive/marx/works/1844/manuscripts/wages.htm.

Maslach, C. and Jackson, S.E. (1982) Burnout in health professions: a social psychological analysis. In G.S. Saders and J. Suis (eds) *Social Psychology of Health and Illness*. Mahwah, NJ: Lawrence Erlbaum Associates.

McCann, C.M., Beddoe, E. McCormick, K., Huggard, P. Kedge, S., Adamson, C. and Huggard, J. (2013) Resilience in the health professions: a review of recent literature. *International Journal of Wellbeing* 3(1): 60–81.

Menzies, I.E.P. (1960) A case study in the functioning of social systems as a defence against anxiety: a report on a study of the nursing service of a general hospital. *Human Relations* 13: 95–121.

O'Driscoll, M., Allan, H.T. and Smith P. (2010) Still looking for leadership – who is responsible for student nurses' learning in practice? *Nurse Education Today* 30(3): 212–218.

Porter, S. (2003) *Flesh in the Age of Reason*. London: Allen Lane.

Proctor, S. (2000) *Caring for Health*. London: Macmillan.

Rafferty, A.M. (1996) *The Politics of Nursing Knowledge*. London: Routledge.

Rutter, M. (2012) Resilience as a dynamic concept. *Development and Psychopathology* 24: 335–344.

Smith, P. (1992) *The Emotional Labour of Nursing: How Nurses Care*. Basingstoke: Palgrave Macmillan.

Smith, P. (2012) *The Emotional Labour of Nursing Revisited: Can Nurses Still Care?* 2nd edition. Basingstoke: Palgrave Macmillan.

Smith, P. (2013) Counter the scapegoating and show the public you still care. Available at: www.nursingtimes.net/nursing-practice/clinical-zones/practice-nursing/counter-the-scapegoating-and-show-the-public-you-still-care/5054842.article.

Snowden, A., Stenhouse, R., Young, J., Carver, H. and Brown, N. (2014) The relationship between emotional intelligence, previous caring experience and mindfulness in student nurses and midwives: a cross sectional analysis. *Nurse Education Today* 35(1): 152–158.

Stayt, C.L. (2009) Death, empathy and self-preservation: the emotional labour of caring for families of the critically ill in adult intensive care. *Journal of Clinical Nursing* 18: 1267–1275.

Theodosius, C. (2008) *Emotional Labour in Health Care: The Unmanaged Heart of Nursing*. London: Routledge.

Wanous, J.P., Reichers, A.E. and Austin, J. (2000) Cynicism about organizational change: measurement, antecedents, and correlates. *Group and Organisation Management* 25: 132–153.

6

Nursing the body

Helen Allan

Issue

Our issue in this chapter is how students learn to care for the body, to nurse the body, and how sociological theory can help us understand this process. We will start by describing the reality of caring for the body in nursing which we think is often missing from textbooks such as this.

Consider the data extract below from Helen Allan and Pam Smith's field notes from their research into Leadership for Learning. Helen is using participant observation, which meant she worked with the first-year student nurse on a hospital ward during a shift while observing, to gather data. This produced copious amounts of field notes.

Medical ward, 07.45, very busy, linen bags, sheets etc all down the corridor; doctors, nurses darting in and out of bays. Sister greeted me with open arms! 1st year student was working with sister but very busy ward and patients in bay needed full washes/ bedbaths. We set to ...

2nd patient was confused, had kept the bay awake by shouting, smelt of faeces and needed a full bedbath. Student went to gather things we'd need and we started. The woman had a big sacral sore, necrotic and 'dirty' with faeces. The bedbath took about 45 minutes; it was hot, smelly, and difficult to move the woman and the student was unsure of herself. However the woman kept saying thank you and looked better afterwards; she then went on to be incontinent of faeces 10 minutes afterwards. After two more bedbaths including assessing a lady who'd 'gone off' (TIA) and doing a set of observations and calling sister who did a superb mini teaching session, we staggered off to coffee.

What are your reactions to these data? Can you remember the first time you cleaned someone who had been incontinent of faeces and how the smell hit you? Perhaps you couldn't show it but when you went home, did you want to wash to get rid of the smell, imagined or not? How long did it take you to get used to smells like this and the task of washing patients after they had been incontinent? Are there other smells that you still find nauseating or perhaps just off-putting? How would you describe this experience to someone from outside nursing or to another nurse? Would you use the same language?

More than one student nurse has told Helen in personal tutor work how they wash their uniform and themselves almost compulsively after shifts. She wonders whether this is because the work feels dirty, polluting almost, and that the memory hangs around like a bad smell. As we will see in this chapter, some sociological theories around dirty work and stigma might help students learn how to approach such work.

The extract above is also striking because we don't often read about this side of caring for bodies. It's somehow hidden from most textbooks and theories of nursing. Some people seem to suggest we nurse patients almost without physical bodies, so metaphysical is our relationship with our patients meant to be.

Now read Helen's reflections on this experience in her field notes.

> I remarked how tired I felt and joked I wasn't used to hard work. Later I reflected in my field notes that the smell had really bothered me and I wondered why. It hadn't used to bother me when I was nursing full time. Had my defences against smelling been lost somehow?

Helen's reflection after washing a patient's body for the first time in a few years illustrates how we learn as nurses to care for bodies; we build up ways of working with dirt and bodies that help us distance ourselves from the reality of this work. Such work is also stigmatising in many societies. Helen's reflection also reminds us that being intimate with patients can be difficult, stressful even, for them as well as us.

This chapter considers what caring for bodies is like and what sociologists have to say about nursing the body.

Chapter outline

This chapter is divided into three broad sections:

- Subjectivity
  - Nursing knowledge, women's knowledge
- The body and nursing care
  - Disciplining the body
  - Basic nursing (bodily) care
  - The medical model of nursing
  - Embodiment and nursing
  - Dirty work
- Stigma and shame

The delivery of nursing or bedside care is now performed largely by support workers yet such care is or should be supervised by trained nurses and is still called *nursing* care. We have discussed this seeming conundrum by exploring the historical development of nursing care in Chapter 4, in particular considering the question 'what is nursing?' and will look at it in terms of 'delegation' in Chapter 8. In this chapter we will explore nursing and the body, what might be called nursing care of the body undertaken when caring for sick patients, and the stigma associated with care of sick people's bodies and mental health needs (the micro perspective). In this chapter we focus more on the micro sociology of the body and stigma.

But first, a question we need to consider before discussing the body in nursing: what is nursing?

What is nursing?

In Chapter 4 we considered nursing as work by taking a macro perspective to understanding nursing as within the context of work generally and nursing's socio-economic position in comparison to other work; here I wish to discuss nursing work in relation to nursing care of the body by taking a micro approach in terms of sociological theory.

In nursing, the question, 'what is nursing?' has been a constant feature of debates in the media and in the profession since Florence Nightingale wrote *Notes on Nursing: What It Is and What It Is Not* (1860). It is worth quoting from the Introduction to Nightingale's *Notes* because it introduces the issues we address in this chapter:

> The [notes] are meant simply to give hints for thought to women who have personal charge of the health of others. Every woman, or at least almost every woman, in England has, at one time or another of her life, charge of the personal health of somebody, whether child or invalid, in other words, every woman is a nurse. Every day sanitary knowledge, or the knowledge of nursing, or in other words, of how to put the constitution in such a state as that it will have no disease, or that it can recover from disease, takes a higher place. It is recognized as the knowledge which every one ought to have – distinct from medical knowledge, which only a profession can have.

A striking feature of Nightingale's vision of nursing is that she sees it as a vocation as distinct from medical (professional) knowledge. It is knowledge which she nevertheless considers a cut above everyday care of the sick; nursing relies on, in her terms, sanitary knowledge.

Of course several important people at the same time as Nightingale did not agree with her view that nursing was a vocation (see Chapter 4). But Nightingale's ideas and her assertion that 'nursing is the knowledge everyone ought to have as distinct from medical knowledge, which only a profession can have', is an idea that is still popular today.

As a student nurse in the twenty-first century, you might not agree that 'every woman is a nurse', especially if you're a man. Nightingale's *gendered* view of nursing and caring might seem outdated to us today. However, her statement 'every woman is a nurse' has had a huge influence on how nursing is viewed by both medicine, the public and policy-makers, and continues to affect nursing's status as professional work.

We considered in Chapter 4 that nursing is gendered work and this stems directly from the development of nursing in the UK and USA under the influence of Nightingale. What is overlooked is that other religions such as Islam have also encouraged the development of a female-only nursing workforce.

As a result of the gendered nature of nursing, certain feminine attributes have become associated with nurses including subjectivity.

Subjectivity and nursing

We've already mentioned feminine attributes such as nurturing, caring, domesticity and submissiveness but we can also include subjectivity, irrationality, feeling or emotionality. And above all nursing has been associated with caring for the body, which was considered dirty, immoral and polluting.

What does subjectivity mean?

We introduced the concept of subjectivity in Chapter 1 when we discussed micro sociology. We said that it was the study of individual experience. A fuller definition is helpful here: 'Subjectivity relates to consciousness, agency, personhood, reality, and truth (Dillon, 2010). Or more simply, 'judgment based on individual personal impressions and feelings and opinions rather than external facts' (www.vocabulary.com/dictionary/subjectivity). Subjectivity explains why one person likes a painting and another hates it.

Micro-sociological theories draw on all three definitions. In this section, however, we want to add to our discussion in Chapter 1 on subjectivity by drawing on feminist theory to show how women's subjectivity and therefore (by default because nursing emerged in the nineteenth and twentieth centuries as a women's profession), nurses' subjectivity, have been devalued as legitimate forms of knowledge over time. We suggest that nursing, through being associated with the feminine and women, was consequently associated with forms of knowledge that were devalued by men, medicine and society in general. These alternative forms of knowledge were seen increasingly as *unscientific*. Nursing knowledge, like nursing, was invisible and perhaps remains so to this day.

Nursing knowledge, women's knowledge

It has been said that:

> Nursing has a distinct knowledge base which is not grounded in empirco-analytic science and its methodology but which stems from the lived experiences of nurses as women and nurses involved in caring relationship with their clients. (Hagell, 1989: 226)

Feminist theories explore multiple realities and subjectivities, which include women's excluded knowledge and subjectivities, that is those of black women, disabled women, lesbians. This is called standpoint epistemology, described by among others

Hilary Rose (born 1935). For feminists it is not just a question of acknowledging women's knowledge but making their contribution to social life visible. British sociologist Ann Oakley (born 1944) made this point some time ago (1984) when she asserted that there was a need to make nursing work as women's work visible. Other feminists wished to go further than acknowledging and valuing women's knowledge; they argued that women's knowledge could provide a more adequate understanding for social life then masculine forms of knowledge.

> Masculinist knowledge takes the form of a peculiar emphasis on the domains of cognitive and objective rationality ... and in dichotomous partitioning of the social and natural worlds. It is this masculinist knowledge which has produced today's deadly culture of science and technology and which seeks to relegate women and women's knowledge to the realm of nature. (Rose, 1986: 162)

In Chapter 2, we gave an illustration of how nursing has been dominated by medical knowledge. According to some feminist theories, this scientific knowledge is, as Rose argues, seen as masculine or masculinist. Now read the case study in the box below.

Scenario 6.1

An ethnographic study of sexual rehabilitation in oncology found that women's sexual lives after their radiotherapy and chemotherapy were seldom asked about in follow-up appointments in oncology outpatients. The interviewees included oncology staff, women and their partners.

In the quote below, the male research fellow describes the difficulty of talking about sexuality in a busy oncology follow-up clinic.

> I think in some ways in a busy clinic that's important because it's got to be about the disease and very often, in terms of psychosocial issues, in terms of chronic side-effects I would feel there should be more of an emphasis upon late side-effects, sexual and whatever others. In terms of psychosocial issues, often the doctor is a poor person, or the worst person you could talk to about, because certainly there isn't an appreciation of issues like that, apart from referral on to someone else. [Male clinician] (White et al., 2013: 192)

The point we want to make here is that masculinist knowledge grounded in science and an understanding of *disease* is inadequate to understand women's experiences. As this male clinician says, 'the doctor is the worst person you [women] could talk to'. Someone else, a referral as he puts it, is needed to appreciate *psychosocial* issues or, for our purpose, women's subjectivities.

Interestingly, what this research quote shows is that 'the comprehensive study and practice of sexual rehabilitation in oncology requires a synthesis of both biomedical and social constructionist [sociological theory] perspectives in order to capture the complex, subjective and embodied nature of the female sexual response in both health and illness' (White et al., 2013: 194).

The body and nursing care

So what insights can sociological theories offer us to help us understand the body in nursing, or nursing care of patients' bodies? We will draw on Michel Foucault's work on discourse and disciplinary practices to explore the body and nursing care. But first we should say that Foucault (1926–1984) was one of the first sociologists to turn his attention to the physical side of our social lives; that is, how our social (and psychological) worlds are intimately connected to our sense of our own bodies and our physical selves, or our embodied selves. But more of that later. For now we will consider Foucault's ideas on disciplining bodies through disciplinary practices.

Disciplining the body

Foucault's theory of the body (which is broadly social constructionist) has been used to understand women's experiences of sexuality. In Chapter 1, we considered social constructionism by introducing Berger and Luckmann's *The Social Construction of Reality*, which was one of the earlier social constructionist theories. We will now consider Foucault's writings on the body as he can offer a way of understanding the critiques of subjectivity – what we have called here anti-subjectivity.

Foucault was a French philosopher rather than a sociologist. His writings have been influential in sociology because he deals with the same difficult questions as sociologists: questions about human behaviour, agency, structures and systems. He is, like Weber, who we introduced in Chapter 1, interested in rationality and bureaucracy, and how each controls individual agency and leaves little room for subjectivity. He thought of societies as systems where individuals were influenced or perhaps constrained to behave not from subjectivity or agency but from *disciplinary practices and discourses*. For Foucault (1979) discourses were overarching systems of meaning that include language, social practices, rituals and social relations. The target of discourses is the individual, the subject or, for our purposes, the patient or the nurse.

His view was that from the seventeenth to the nineteenth century, institutions increased their control over the body through institutional practices such as censuses or institutions, the asylum, the prison, the clinic and the state (Foucault, 1973). These practices were legitimised through discourses, Foucault drew attention to how society (developing capitalist societies) 'evolved to make control and regulation of the body, and hence the subjugation of individuals and society, a core preoccupation' through rational surveillance (Dillon, 2010: 351) As Dillon says, while Foucault didn't consider the gendered control of bodies, he does make us think in a new way about the body and the social processes through which we control the body.

Rational surveillance was a disciplinary practice exerted on the body to produce *docile bodies*. Foucault thought that modern society reins in, monitors and disciplines the body in parts through institutions as much as by individuals themselves.

So the discourse of health promotion is a good way to understand Foucault's view of rational surveillance working to discipline bodies. Schooling is another form of rational surveillance where our children learn to sit still, attend and become good citizens or perhaps subjects. In the prison, he found another example of disciplining bodies to make well-behaved citizens.

Foucault's work has been used by nurses writing about the body, including Jocalyn Lawler (born 1949) who wrote about the 'problem of the body for nursing' by which she meant that the body was the focus of nursing practice, yet it is not spoken about and devalued when it is referred to. This is because caring for the body is 'dirty' and devalued work associated with women's domestic work; it is literally dirty, dealing with blood, faeces, urine and in extreme cases, for example dealing with an aborted foetus, it is taboo. In fact, Lawler suggests that nursing 'involves crossing social boundaries, breaking taboos and doing things for people which they would normally do' (1991: 32).

Reflection 6.1

- What sorts of tasks in caring for patients' bodies have you undertaken?
- How did performing these intimate, bodily tasks make you feel?
- Did you feel slightly awkward and, if so, why?
- What do you think about Lawler's theory of 'crossing social boundaries'?

Lawler calls her theorising of the bodywork in nursing practice *somology*; by which she means working with the object body (the material or objective body) *and* the subjective body (the lived body). Meutzal expresses this integration of the objective and subjective body as the potential of nursing the body as 'closeness at a physical, psychological and spiritual level' (1988: 98). Somology draws on Foucauldian theory to integrate his insights into the disciplining of the objective body yet retain a lived subjective body. As we shall see later, somology may not capture the majority of nursing care that nurses deliver, which is subject to the constraints of the health-care system and frequently is arranged around medical tasks, task allocation and along rigid hierarchical lines. Of course at different points in time and in some fields more than others, closeness as Meutzal and Lawler describe may be possible such as in the *new nursing* in nursing development units in the 1990s in the UK, described by Jan Savage in her book *Nursing Intimacy* (1995). In other body work, such as prostitution or beauty therapy, think epilation, intimacy or closeness aren't always what the client or the body worker wishes to achieve. A further criticism of somological or phenomenological approaches in nursing is that they tend to restrict the analysis of power in nursing relationships with patients, and importantly with medicine, which affects the delivery of nursing care.

Two other nurses who are also sociologically minded and have written about the body are Cheek and Porter, who argue that Foucault's idea of *discourse* offers a way of thinking about power relations that, in turn, structure nurses' daily working lives and the nursing practices they either chose or are required to practise

(Cheek and Porter, 1997). There are, of course, many discourses, each articulating a distinct disciplinary practice of care. We will consider three disciplinary practices that are contained in nursing discourses: basic nursing (bodily) care, medical nursing model and embodiment in nursing.

Basic nursing (bodily) care

Nursing care of bodies is integral to nursing yet it is still frequently referred to as *basic nursing care*; we shall suggest why later in this chapter. Of course in more recent nursing curricula, basic care is now called fundamentals or essentials of care. But however one labels the work, nursing care of bodies still involves work that is devalued, lower paid and socially unacceptable to talk openly about. In some circumstances, it is socially taboo, such as in bowel care, care of fungating wounds or certain forms of disability.

Scenario 6.2

Brown et al.'s (2008) paper on doctors' and nurses' approaches to infection control policies is an interesting case study. It deals with the everyday issue of infection control, which we probably all take for granted and has become part and parcel of our everyday practice. In this paper the authors discuss the macro policy of infection control in the context of medical staff breaches of that policy as an example of taboo about the control of dirt in hospitals.

As the infection control manager says, trying to get doctors as well as nurses to clean their hands thoroughly has been an uphill struggle:

So I've worked very hard, passionately, with one of the doctors in the medical school, so that the medical students have to undergo a hand hygiene examination ... just like the nurses have had to do for many, many years.

But it is still difficult to change medical practice it appears, as one of the descriptions of the doctors in the hospital where the research was undertaken is 'delinquent doctors', and the nurse managers want to do anything they can to 'get their scores up' to show they are complying with hospital policy on infection control.

What this research shows is how more widely in the hospital dirt becomes a marker of poor practice, of breaching boundaries and spreading infection; rather like breaking a taboo feels perhaps.

But there are other taboos in nursing. Nursing care of the body involves touch and intimacy; students and nurses entering the profession encounter nursing care of the body with their own cultural beliefs and experience about appropriate behaviours when caring for others' bodies. Touch and intimacy, which are integral to nursing care of bodies are in this sense socially and culturally constructed. Students therefore may have to work to overcome previously held beliefs and even taboos to deliver bodily or intimate care. Read the box below and consider your reactions to Lawler's writing on sexuality.

Reflection 6.2

Lawler (1991) pays particular attention to sexuality because the majority of nurses are females making it difficult for them to understand the male patient's body experiences. Male sexuality says Lawler is focused on the genitals and certain care activities will be more sensitive to female nurses and male patients.

Think of giving catheter care to a patient of the opposite sex. How do you feel? Embarrassed? Shy? Shamed?

In Crossan and Mathew's study (2013) students clearly expressed that they found caring for patients of the opposite sex difficult, embarrassing and shameful; and that they were unprepared and unsupported for this aspect of their work.

How prepared were you for caring for a patient's sexuality?

Another factor to affect whether a student felt embarrassed was age. The older the patient, the less embarrassment was experienced. However, this age difference and the lack of embarrassment meant that the students described their care as depersonalised or desexualised because they did not identify with the patient.

Think about where you have noticed nurses or other healthcare staff who approach patients in a depersonalised way. Consider what might be prompting them to do this.

Or have you ever caught yourself feeling detached or treating a patient in a depersonalised manner? Why? What was going on at the time to make this happen?

You might like to consider how detachment can be a good way to care for patients.

As a follow-up to this activity, you might like to read Allan and Barber (2005) and reflect on the material in Chapter 5, 'Caring, face-work and nursing'.

Caring for a patient's body also grants the nurse privileges in their lived experiences of nursing and in their relationships with patients (Lawler, 1991; Savage, 1995; Grant et al., 2005). Even giving a patient a wash or adjusting an incontinence sheath entails intimate touch and an invasion of privacy which in ordinary social circumstances would not be tolerated. As we've seen in Chapter 5, Menzies (1970) argues that nurses deal with the extraordinary in their everyday work; she suggested that nursing work is emotionally charged because it deals with tasks that are by 'ordinary standards' distasteful, disgusting and frightening. Nevertheless, for both nurse and patient, this disgust needs to be overcome, and the intimacy and breach of privacy entailed in giving nursing or bodily care needs to be tolerated.

Menzies suggests that nursing has over time built up protocols to manage the discomfort of their role, to manage the disgust, in caring for the body. She argued that task allocation arranged along lines of hierarchy and seniority, an integral part of the medical model of nursing (see below), was one very effective way that disgust was managed in nursing patients and delivering intimate care. Task allocation where the junior nurses washed patients, someone a bit more senior did the observations, someone else even more senior delivered medications and the ward sister supervised the discharges and admissions was a way of distancing the nurse from the discomfort and even disgust. This system relied on a hierarchy of tasks and a hierarchy of nursing staff. Of course, you might say that as a student nurse at the beginning of the twenty-first century patients are nursed so differently that this analysis of nursing is outdated and even far-fetched. But consider the research data in the box below.

Scenario 6.3

Observation notes/medical ward/site A:

I arrive at 07.30 and no one about as all staff in office at handover. I wait. They all come out. No one comes to ask me who I am. Students stream into kitchen and start breakfasts; staff nurses start drugs and bed state ... after introducing myself, I work with students to do breakfasts. After we finish, I ask 'what next?' 'Beds' and so we go to do beds ... it feels as things haven't changed since the 1970s when I started training! There's certainly no patient allocation to the students; we all pitch in.

Excerpt from Report to the General Nursing Council of England & Wales on the Leadership for Learning Project (Allan et al., 2008)

Helen and Pam were the researchers on the Leadership for Learning project (Allan et al., 2008) and in these observation notes of one observation on a medical ward in an acute NHS trust, Helen reflects on how easy it was to fit into the routine and how familiar the task allocation appeared. On further reflection while writing this chapter, the division of labour along hierarchical lines as suggested by Menzies is quite clear in this data extract.

But what is the purpose of this nursing approach to nursing the body? That might seem like an oxymoronic question but consider that in many parts of the world patients are cared for by their relatives yet that has never been the case in the UK. Why? Perhaps, as Nightingale argued, it was woman's work, and therefore thought to be natural; or perhaps it was difficult to develop nursing beyond the traditional domestic roles in a time when women's roles outside the home were restricted, as we argue in Chapter 4. However, Lawler and others have suggested that the traditional nursing approach to nursing care of the body is a form of disciplinary practice; that is, we keep patients in a passive position through nursing them in beds, asking them to remove their clothes, keep to a ward timetable and generally behave.

Reflection 6.3

Read Felicity Stockwell's seminal research report *The Unpopular Patient*. In it she shows how nurses use various tactics to manage patients' behaviour
   The whole report can be downloaded from this link: www2.rcn.org.uk/__data/assets/pdf_file/0005/235508/series_1_number_2.pdf.
   How accurate do you think her observations of the interactions between patients and nursing staff were?
   Can you think of patients who might have been unpopular in clinical areas where you've been a student?
   Most of the comments expressed by nurses about patients appear to concern behaviours; there are some references to nursing care of the body: patients being unpopular if they were heavy or they obstructed nurses from giving care. Why do you think this is?

What Stockwell's research findings suggest is that, despite the aspiration to care in Florence Nightingale's *Notes on Nursing* and subsequently, there is clearly a lack of caring when nursing patients. Nurses actually demand certain types of behaviour: if they wish to be cared for, they need to behave and nurses will sanction patients if they step out of line. In its worst form, this is perhaps what was seen at Winterbourne View (see 'Going further' for link to YouTube news reports into the enquiry of the Winterbourne care home). Of course, none of this is explicit although the signs you see in hospitals saying you will be prosecuted if you are rude or aggressive to hospital staff is one way this form of implicit expectation of patient and family behaviour has changed over the years. Nursing care of the body, including physical care, interactions, intimacy and ward routine, is therefore a form of disciplinary practice buried within a discourse of care.

The medical model of nursing

We suggested in an earlier section that what constitutes nursing care has always been contested. The nursing care of the body is equally contested and there are different ways of thinking or conceptualising the body in nursing. We've suggested that Foucault's ideas around disciplining the body could be applied to how basic nursing care or the fundamentals of care are delivered. We've introduced an alternative view, that of Lawler's theory of somology and nursing; that is, the idea of the lived body for both patient and nurse and being attentive to the lived body in caring for patients. We shall address this in more detail shortly in a section on embodiment. We've also drawn your attention to touch, intimacy and emotions when caring for the bodies of patients and, importantly, taboos around the body. The medical model of nursing, where nursing is broken down into tasks based on the parts of the body, has probably been the most dominant model of nursing since Nightingale's time. Indeed, as we have suggested, task allocation is still entrenched in nursing in the acute setting (Allan et al., 2011). We have suggested that task allocation may be one way nursing has developed to manage the distaste of nursing the incontinent, the hurting or the (literally) dirty body.

In another study, this time in New Zealand, Grant et al. (2005) argue that 'Intimate bodily care is not only contestable … [it] is also often a taken-for-granted aspect of nursing students' preparation for the clinical setting'.

Student nurses in Grant et al. argue that the embarrassment Lawler talks about is rarely addressed in nursing education and that as a consequence they are unprepared for caring for the body in intimate ways. They learn pretty quickly, probably like you, that there is a dominant model of caring for the body in nursing that is called the medical model.

Grant et al. go on to argue that the dominant model of nursing care is the scientific medical discourse of care. By this we mean that nursing care was derived originally from 'medical orders' where the doctor gave instructions for care of a patient, including how to nurse them, to put them in the best state for the medical intervention to work. As the Nightingale pledge, which American nurses swear to uphold on qualifying, describes it, 'I will endeavour to aid the physician in his work'. Because nurses worked so closely with doctors, aiding the physicians, they developed good knowledge of bodily disease based on biomedical knowledge, associated symptoms and appropriate treatments so they could support the doctor and 'cure' the patient. They were effectively the doctor's *handmaiden*.

In medicine the patient is made up of biological and physiological parts and is essentially a passive object – think of Parsons' sick-role model which we introduced in Chapter 1. The work of nursing in medically led settings consists of a clearly delineated set of procedures, to be undertaken rigorously and supervised by a nurse directly accountable to the doctor. Hence the importance of having the consultant's name over in-patient beds in hospitals and the ward round where the nurse in charge is asked to account for the care of patients to *their* consultant. Lawler described these procedures as 'typically procedural, objective, if not objectifying and clinical'. Consider another extract from the observation notes of another research study Helen has been involved with.

Scenario 6.4

Observation notes/day surgery/site B:

I sit and observe a bay's activities. First the students and healthcare assistants (HCAs) 'do' the breakfasts, then the HCAs give out bowls to those patients who need them and they and the student makes beds. The staff nurse comes in and starts the drugs.

Extract from Report into Newly Qualified Nurses' Delegation to and Supervision of Health Care Assistants 2014 http://www2.surrey.ac.uk/fhms/research/centres/crnme/currentactivity/AaRK%20project/aark-summary-report.pdf.

In this extract from her observation notes, Helen observes that the tasks in the bay where six patients sleep and spend their days are divided along quite clear lines which were repeated across different clinical areas in three hospitals. After handover between shifts *which the assistants did not attend*, the staff worked on specific parts of the patient's care: the staff nurse on the medications, the assistant and student on the more intimate/basic aspects of the care including the bed making. This meant that the nurse could be giving medication without knowing anything about the patient's mobility, skin integrity or just how s/he felt. While the assistant could be giving body care without knowing anything about the patient's condition. They were each caring for parts of the patient's body without any knowledge of the part as a whole.

Of course, Nightingale considered that nursing alongside and directed by medicine was a higher calling, or vocation, but does the medical model still carry higher status for some nurses?

In a study into the skills and aptitudes men and women might bring to nursing, Simpson (2011: 386) found men preferred diagnostics and the medical model of nursing. She argues that the female nurses she interviewed had a 'wry acceptance of hands-on care of other people's bodies as women's work' and commented 'yeah the guys, I must say, do like an emergency – you won't find many on the wards changing bedpans for long!' Simpson calls this the flight from the body by men and argues that caring for bodies was seen as devalued work, suitable for women and difficult to reconcile with beliefs about masculinities. Simpson's findings are seen in other work in this area which investigates gendered hierarchies of nursing work.

While this talk of nursing history and the emphasis on task allocation and caring for patients' bodies as body parts may seem excessive, take some time to read Helmstadter's account of Florence Nightingale's Scutari nursing experience (in Nelson and Rafferty (2010) in 'Going further'). It will help you understand the often unequal relationship between medicine and nursing and why the struggle for nursing with full professional status has not been entirely successful.

Why do we distinguish between the basic model of (bodily) care and the medical model of care? Neither of them offer an appreciation of the physical body as both seek to either compartmentalise it into medical tasks or deny the reality of the incontinent body.

The last disciplinary practice we will discuss here is embodiment – a much more recent approach to nursing the body which acknowledges the leaky, incontinent and at times polluting body.

Embodiment and nursing

So much of how we think about the body, and nursing the body, has been shaped by the sixteenth-century French philosopher René Descartes (1596–1650). Have a look at this YouTube clip (www.youtube.com/watch?v=0A6UKoMcE10) for some more information about Descartes' Philosophy.

Descartes believed that we were made up of our bodies and our minds, and for him the mind was the key to ourselves – 'je pense, donc je suis' (I think, therefore I am) – but later philosophers believed that mind and body cannot be separated. This way of thinking about the body is called Cartesian duality; dualism is the idea that the mind and body are two quite different and opposing things. This Cartesian view of the world underpins medical thought, the view that a body can be studied separately in parts. This is evident in how medical specialisms are delineated: plastics, cancer, psychiatry, medicine, surgery, neurology, endocrinology and so on.

Embodiment is very different to Cartesian thought and medicine because it assumes that the mind and body are connected, intertwined and real to each other; we live in our minds and through our bodies (Wilde, 1999). This way of thinking comes from phenomenology again (see Lawler above); we are embodied beings and no part can be separated from the rest.

Consider this quote from Goyder's account of caring for patients with Alzheimer's disease:

> I had never been so conscious of people's bodies as when I began working in nursing homes. Patients, especially those with dementias were often handled without any awareness or consideration of their 'selfness', handled as if they were bodies and nothing else. ... they [patients] were touched, handled, repositioned, toileted and so on constantly throughout the day and [have] no choice over whether they were touched. Many became limp, immobilized, refusing to move themselves or help in any way even if they could. Refusing also to speak, these patients began to seem like heavy lumps of flesh, nothing else – all body. (2001: 123–124)

This quote conveys the complex ways in which, as Lawler says, 'human beings are as much embodied as we are enselved'; that is, who we are is as much our mind as our body. Read the box below and consider how technological advances separate our bodies and therefore our sense of embodiment from ourselves.

Scenario 6.5

To illustrate embodiment in everyday nursing practice, Mary Wilde (1999) gives the example of a patient with an intravenous pump. She asks what effect does the physical technology have on the patient as a whole? A patient can no more separate themselves from the pump as they can from other parts of who they are.

You might like to read Wilde's paper 'Why embodiment now?' (see 'Going further') as she gives a good overview of the history of the body and its implications for nursing. She has some good examples of how recently an embodied understanding of the body has begun to influence practice.

Think about asthma patients and how we teach them to control their breathing through mindfulness. Or how patients with long-term catheters might be taught to pay attention to their bodies in a more embodied fashion to prevent urinary tract infections.

Have you seen other ways in which you've noticed embodied care of patients?

Lawler argues that our sense of our bodies has become increasingly separated from a) our sense of who we are and b) our sense of having whole bodies rather than body parts. So the patients in Goyder's quote, having no control over their care, were treated as bodies rather than selves, and then they took themselves out of their care so that Goyder says they became '*all body*'. Academic disciplines of the body tend to add to this sense of parts rather than the whole body, for example psychology, biology and chemistry.

However, when nurses care for patients' bodies, when they do the caring work on bodies, is it just that – *work* – or does the nurse have to care for her patients as well as do the caring? Can the nurse and patient achieve 'closeness at a physical, psychological and spiritual level' in the caring act as Meutzal suggests? (See our discussion on emotions in Chapter 5.)

Wolkowitz (2002), a sociologist who studies caring in care homes, suggests that we should distinguish between a) instrumental caring work which is the task, and b) the gift of care which is what writers like Lawler and Meutzal are talking about. She argues that somewhere the reality of caring work has got lost in the phenomenology of caring to the detriment of awareness of women's work experiences. That is, we are in danger of forgetting how difficult, messy and demanding and low paid caring work is. Wolkowitz suggests that 'elevating the psychological, so that in contrasts the body becomes, mindlessness or mechanical response' has, ironically, replicated the Cartesian splitting of mind–body. Wolkowitz also argues, like White et al. above, that the links between our social lives and our existence as embodied human beings as well as the physical, biological determinants of our lives, need to be integrated into a social model of the body, one that includes the messy, leaky and smelly body.

In the next section, having discussed three disciplinary practices in nursing, we will consider the reality of women's paid caring work, or *dirty work*.

Dirty and devalued work

Repeated studies of nursing in Western societies have shown that nursing care of the body is considered dirty and, consequently, devalued.

Now consider the activity in the box below.

Reflection 6.4

Do you think a different status is placed on the different roles associated with the clean tasks of nursing (medicines, administration) and the dirty tasks (washing patients, changing bed linen, emptying urinary bags and bedpans) at handover.

And now think of which tasks you value more highly? Is it emptying a patient's bedpan or arranging a patient's discharge?

Which areas of nursing are generally more highly valued than others? Is older care, where there is a much higher level of 'dirty' tasks, valued above intensive care or cardiac care?

If you do feel that some nursing tasks and some areas of nursing are seen either by you or your mentors as higher status than others, this should not surprise you. As long ago as 1953, a researcher called Goddard found that nursing could be defined as technical (medications), affective (listening) and basic work (washing patients, emptying bedpans). In subsequent work by nurse researchers Fretwell (1982) and Melia (1982), it was found that nurses and nursing students valued these components of nursing work, technical, affective and basic, differently; each was assigned low or high status. The highest status being given to technical tasks. The students who Melia interviewed described affective nursing as 'not really nursing'. Smith (1992) goes on to argue that there are differences between a 'professional rhetoric of caring and nurses' own work priorities'. These differences may be because the experience of learning for student nurses is not always in itself a caring process (see Chapter 5). You might consider the idea of nursing the body as dirty work rather exaggerated but consider the words used by students in a study by Crossnan and Mathew describing nursing body care included embarrassment, discomfort, shame, awkwardness and inappropriate. Despite these strong words which suggest that learning to give intimate body care is challenging for students, they also described such care as a necessary part of nursing and the requirement for them to learn to be professional: 'it's my professional duty to look after the hygiene needs of my patient' (third-year student, Crossan and Mathew, 2013: 319).

A different study by Grant et al. (2005) also found that students experienced discomfort, embarrassment and distress at handling the body and delivering intimate care for patients.

In her analysis of nursing cross culturally, Wolf (1996: 27) argues that nursing is dirty work and that 'those [nurses/midwives] who perform dirty work are soiled by association'. Nursing tasks that would be seen as dirty would include washing patients' bodies, dealing with elimination and other matters such as blood, sputum, wound dressings and exudate. In discussing the dirt of nursing tasks, sociologists have drawn on Douglas' (1966) discussion of the ritual separation of dirty and clean in many cultures; the clean being associated with the sacred and dirty with the profane.

Twigg (2000: 408) has used Lawler's work to study the giving of care as dirty work. Twigg suggests that care includes touching, cleaning and comforting the patient (or elderly care resident) in ways that 'violate cultural codes of disgust at bodily functions and fluids and the avoidance of close contact'. This is a particular issue for Western societies where the body is seen as intimate and private and bodily fluids and secretions as polluting and taboo (Douglas, 1966). Such dirty work, as it becomes known, is then hidden from others and the doing of it penalises those who perform it. Those who do dirty work are predominantly women and the work is devalued and poorly paid.

Actually this association of nursing with polluting work can be seen in Islamic cultures and may be one reason why recruiting Islamic students into nursing is challenging cross-culturally. In a PhD study supervised by Helen and Pam, the student, herself a practising Muslim nurse, found that some newly qualified Saudi nurses in Saudi Arabia did not wish to continue as nurses because it is seen as work that pollutes.

In our last section, we link the work we have presented on disciplining practices in nursing, the 'basic' care model, the medical model and the embodiment model, and the idea of nursing the body as dirty work with a sociological theory we considered in Chapter 1, ethnomethodological approaches and, in particular, Goffman's theory of stigma.

Stigma

In Chapter 1, we suggested there that stigma is frequently experienced along with shame. For example, we have suggested malignant fungating wounds, sexual health and cancer are stigmatising conditions along with many forms of disability. Here we draw on Goffman's ideas of stigma as rule breaking and the experience of shame to discuss nursing's dirty work and the consequences of nursing's association with *dirt*.

In Chapter 1, we suggested that stigma is a process where society labels a person with certain conditions (medical, social or psychological) as shameful, polluting and deviant; they evoked feelings of disgust and/or shame because they broke expectations of social norms. People including the affected person assigned a negative meaning to the person concerned. This negative evaluation may be 'felt' or 'enacted'. A felt negative evaluation refers to the shame associated with having a condition and to the fear of being discriminated against on the grounds of imputed inferiority or social unacceptability (Fitzpatrick et al., 1984). An enacted negative evaluation refers to actual discrimination of this kind.

Stigma can lead to feelings of guilt, shame and spoiled identity. Stigma and shame we argue here is attached to nursing care of bodies because such work breaks social barriers and taboos and is thought of as socially and physically polluting. Therefore those who perform such work, nurses and support staff, are stigmatised and shamed by the work. Please note that this does not mean they *themselves* feel ashamed, but that the work is shaming in the eyes of others. As just one recent example, Simpson (2011) in her study of nursing as gendered work found that women (nurse interviewees) referred to such work (nursing care) as 'dirty, drudgery, hard slog and mind-numbing'.

As a consequence of delivering stigmatised work and feeling shame at breaking taboos, nurses distance themselves from the act of caring and value higher-status tasks such as medications. One sociological explanation of this state of affairs is given by Carpenter (1995).

Carpenter (1995) argues that nursing's association with medicine led to the emergence of a technology and a science of caring that focused on new roles and tasks (often delegated from medicine) rather than activities of daily living and this shift gave it a form of social control and professional status (as we have argued in this chapter). Carpenter argues that caring activities were never at the heart of nursing. Over time, nursing has given caring away to enrolled nurses, student nurses and, more recently, healthcare assistants through carefully delineating a hierarchy of tasks and technologies over which nurses retain control; there are also some tasks such as assessment that nursing has not given away in a professional strategy to differentiate nursing from '*not-nursing*'. I have called this process nursing practice's uncoupling from caring activities while retaining a claim to the philosophy of caring. It is a process commented on by overseas trained nurses recruited to work in the UK.

Stigma is also experienced by patients with certain conditions and by association therefore with the nurse who cares for them. I recommended you read Felicity Stockwell's short research report *The Unpopular Patient* (1972), mentioned earlier in this chapter. You might like to read the short section on page 68 where she talks about patients who are unpopular bearing stigma due to their illness. And lastly, complete this activity.

Reflection 6.5

Think of patients who are unpopular and whether they might carry a stigma.

What has been your reaction to patients with stigmatised conditions such as colostomies, disfiguring surgery, fungating tumours or wounds, burns, exudating wounds, bowel disorders?

How have other people reacted and has there been gossiping? Can you see any behaviours the ward team you were working in at the time shared with Stockwell's ward teams?

Was anything done to support you or the patient in coping with this stigmatising condition?

Chapter summary

It is often said that 'nursing is a practical skill that must be learned by doing it', implying it is a basic skill that you learn on the job; in fact, all of us at some point during our time in nurse education, have had practising nurses say to us that not only is nursing care practical (meaning basic), it doesn't need education (meaning a degree) and nurses don't want to touch patients. We see this as a simplistic argument which is frequently articulated in the media where the effects of structural conditions are largely ignored. Instead the blame for poor nursing care is laid at individual nurses' feet or perhaps nurse education or whomsoever the current whipping boy is. In contrast, we have argued in this book that structural factors such as the sexual and gendered division of labour, the lack of professional status of nursing and its early origins in the reform of nursing in the UK and USA shaped nursing work and its characterisation as an extension of women's domestic work.

In this chapter we've suggested that as well as the structural factors we've discussed in other chapters, nursing was associated with the female and all that represented in nineteenth-century societies in Western Europe and the USA as well as in established Islamic societies; that is, it was associated with feminine attributes and activities such as caring for the sick patient and the body. A quote from Nightingale's *Notes on Nursing* is illustrative of this association. Many people believed nursing was a 'silly display of feminine sensibilities'; that is, it was natural work for women. But it was also deeply *dirty* work which carried a stigma.

Going further

Chapple, A. (2004) Stigma, shame, and blame experienced by patients with lung cancer: qualitative study. *British Medical Journal* 328: 1470–1476.

Helmstadter, C. (2010) Navigating the political straits in the Crimean War. In S. Nelson and A.M. Rafferty (eds) *Notes on Nightingale*. pp. 28–54. Available at: http://digitalcommons.ilr.cornell.edu/cgi/viewcontent.cgi?article=1060&context=books.

Lupton, D. and Schmied, V. (2013) Splitting bodies/selves: women's concepts of embodiment at the moment of birth. *Sociology of Health & Illness* 35(6): 828–841.

Sachs, A. (1988) *The Soft Vengeance of a Freedom Fighter*. (Justice Sachs' response to his loss of an arm and an eye in a terrorist bombing during apartheid in South Africa tells us about he adapted both physically and phenomenologically to his losses.)

Sacks, O. (l984) *A Leg to Stand On*. London: Duckworth. (Oliver Sacks tells us about his mountaineering accident and his phenomenological experience of pain.)

Wilde, M. (1999) Why embodiment now? *Advance in Nursing Science* 22(2): 25–38.

A YouTube video of the press report into poor practices of care of people with learning disability at the Winterbourne View care home: www.youtube.com/watch?v=hhCx3K8XJJM.

References

Allan, H.T. and Barber, D. (2005) Emotion boundary work in advanced fertility nursing roles. *Nursing Ethics* 12(4): 391–400.

Allan, H.T., Smith, P. and O'Driscoll, M. (2008) *GNC Leadership for Learning Research Highlights*. Available at: www.survey.ac.uk/fhms/research/centres/crnme/Completed%20 Projects/Reports/GNC%20main%20report%2022%2005%2008PAS.pdf.

Allan, H.T., Smith, P.A. and O'Driscoll, M. (2011) Experiences of supernumerary status and the hidden curriculum in nursing: a new twist in the theory–practice gap? *Journal of Clinical Nursing* 20: 847–855.

Berger, P.L. and Luckmann, T. (1966) *The Social Construction of Reality. A Treatise on the Sociology of Knowledge*. Garden City, NY: Anchor Books.

Brown, B.J., Crawford, P., Nerlich. B. and Koteyko, N. (2008) The habitus of hygiene: discourses of cleanliness and infection control in nursing work. *Social Science and Medicine* 67(7): 1047–1055.

Carpenter, M. (1995) Doctors and nurses: stereotypes and stereotype change in interprofessional education. *Journal of Interprofessional Care* 9(2): 151–161

Cheek, J. and Porter, S. (1997) Reviewing Foucault: possibilities and problems for nursing and health care. *Nursing Inquiry* 4: 108–119.

Crossan, M. and Mathew, T.K. (2013) Exploring sensitive boundaries in nursing education: attitudes of undergraduate student nurses providing intimate care to patients. *Nurse Education in Practice* 13: 317–322.

Dillon, M. (2010) *Introduction to Sociological Theory: Theorists, Concepts and Their Applicability to the Twenty-First Century*. Chichester: Wiley-Blackwell.

Douglas, M. (1966) *Purity and Danger: An Analysis of Concepts of Pollution and Taboo*. London: Routledge & Kegan Paul.

Fitzpatrick, R., Hinton, J., Newman, S., Scambler, G., Thompson, J. and Scambler, G. (1984) Perceiving and coping with stigmatizing illness. In R. Fitzpatrick, J. Hinton, S. Newman, G. Scambler and J. Thompson (eds) *The Experience of Illness*. London: Tavistock, pp. 203–226.

Foucault, M. (1973) *The Birth of the Clinic*. London: Tavistock.

Foucault, M. (1979) *Discipline and Punish: The Birth of the Prison*. New York: Vintage.

Fretwell, J.E. (1982) *Ward Teaching and Learning: Sister and the Learning Environment*. London: Royal College of Nursing.

Goddard, H.A. (1953) *The Work of Nurses in Hospital Wards: Report of a Job Analysis*. London: Nuffield Provincial Hospitals Trust.

Goyder, J. (2001) *We'll Be Married In Fremantle: Alzheimer's Disease and the Everyday Act of Storying*. Fremantle, Western Australia: Fremantle Arts Centre Press.

Grant, B.M., Giddings, L.S. and Beale, J.E. (2005) Vulnerable bodies: competing discourses of intimate care. *Journal of Nursing Education* 44(11): 498–504.

Hagell, E. (1993) Reproductive technologies and court-ordered obstetrical interventions: the need for a feminist voice in nursing. *Health Care for Women International* 14(1): 77–86.

Hagell, E.I. (1989) Nursing knowledge, women's knowledge: a sociological perspective. *Journal of Advanced Nursing*, 14(3): 226–233.

Lawler, J. (1991) *Behind the Screens: Nursing, Somology and the Problem of the Body*. Melbourne: Churchill Livingstone.

Martin, E. (1987) *The Woman in the Body: A Cultural Analysis of Reproduction*. Boston: Beacon.

Melia, K. (1982) 'Tell it as it is': qualitative methodology and nursing research. *Journal of Advanced Nursing* 7(4): 327–335.

Menzies, I.E.P. (1970) *The Functioning of Social Systems as a Defence Against Anxiety*. London: The Tavistock Institute of Human Relations.

Meutzal, A.P. (1988) Therapeutic nursing. In A. Pearson (ed.) *Primary Nursing: Nursing in the Burford and Oxford Nursing Development Units*. London: Chapman-Hall, pp.89–116.

Nightingale, F. (1860) *Notes on Nursing: What It Is and What It Is Not*. http://digital.library.upenn.edu/women/nightingale/nursing/nursing.html

Oakley, A. (1984) The importance of being a nurse. *Nursing Times* 12 December, 24–27.

Rose, H. (1986) Women's work: women's knowledge. In J. Mitchell and A. Oakley (eds) *What is Feminism?* New York: Pantheon.

Savage, J. (1995) *Nursing Intimacy*. London: Scutari Press.

Simpson, R. (2011) Men discussing women and women discussing men: reflexivity, transformation and gendered practice in the context of nursing care. *Gender, Work & Organisation* 18(4): 377–398.

Smith, P. (1992) *The Emotional Labour of Nursing*. Oxford: Palgrave.

Stockwell, F. (1972) *The Unpopular Patient*. London: Royal College of Nursing.

Twigg, J. (2000) *Bathing: The Body and Community Care*. London: Routledge.

Twigg, J. (2006) The body, gender and caring: work and welfare in Britain and Scandanavia. *Journal of Aging Studies* 18: 59–73.

White, I., Faithfull, S. and Allan, H.T. (2013) The re-construction of women's sexual lives after pelvic radiotherapy: a synthesis of biomedical and sociological perspectives on the study of female sexuality after cancer. *Social Science & Medicine* 76(1): 188–196.

Wilde, M.A. (1999) A phenomenological study of the lived experience of long-term urinary catheterization. Unpublished thesis. Rochester, NY, University of Rochester.

Wolf, Z.R. (1996) Bowel management and nursing's hidden work. *Nursing Times* 92(21): 26–28.

Wolkowitz, C. (2002) The social relations of body work. *Work Employment and Society* 16(3): 497–510.

7

When things go wrong

Daniel Kelly

The issue

In this chapter we will explore why the standard of care that people might expect from health or care services is not always provided. You will be invited to think about clinical situations – such as the one described below – and consider whether sociological insights, especially those from the work of Erving Goffman and Dianne Vaughan, might be helpful in explaining why things can go so badly wrong. We will also discuss recent research carried out by myself and colleagues and encourage you to think about your own role in shaping the culture of your workplaces, and when and how you might consider speaking out.

Consider this extract from the Francis Report (2013):

'We got there about 10 o'clock and I could not believe my eyes. The door was wide open. There were people walking past. Mum was in bed with the cot sides up and she hadn't got a stitch of clothing on. I mean, she would have been horrified. She was completely naked and if I said covered in faeces, she was. It was everywhere. It was in her hair, her eyes, her nails, her hands and all on the cot sides, so she had obviously been trying to lift herself up or move about, because the bed was covered and it was literally everywhere and it was dried. It would have been there a long time, it wasn't new.' (Daughter of a patient quoted in the Mid Staffordshire NHS Foundation Trust Public Inquiry (Francis, 2013))

Reflection 7.1

Before we proceed further you are invited to think about the above extract described by the daughter of an elderly patient. The first question we might ask is, how can this possibly happen? But then we can consider, how does this situation make you feel? How might this woman's daughter react towards those who are responsible for caring for her mother? How would you feel to be a nurse working in this hospital and reading this extract? Finally, and perhaps most importantly, what could we learn from this situation?

Bear your answers to these questions in mind as you read this chapter.

Chapter outline

- Why do things go wrong?
- Workplace cultures and the normalisation of deviance
- Whistleblowing and its alternatives
- When other things go wrong: avoidant leadership and bullying
- Speaking truth to power, and to yourself

Why do things go wrong?

This is the key question for this chapter – and it has relevance to everyone involved in healthcare, including national politicians who decide where and how to invest resources and trust boards and health-service managers who hear about, and who should scrutinise and be accountable for, the services provided to local people.

However, there are also valuable insights that may be drawn from individual clinical examples of care delivery. These will also be shaped by the routines and social practices that govern the way that nurses or other members of the healthcare team are functioning. These routines are powerful and can be difficult to challenge – as we shall see. However, by recognising them you can begin to develop insight into their power and consider whether you can play a role in re-shaping at least part of the culture in which you work. We can also learn from situations outside of health and for this we can consider the lessons from the space shuttle *Challenger* disaster after it exploded soon after launch in 1986. The insights gained thereafter have useful parallels for the National Health Service (NHS) today concerning managerial decision-making and the management of risk.

Scandals in healthcare settings are not new. There have been many over the years and, despite the creation of whistleblowing policies, there is evidence of a gap between the policy in theory, and its practical impact. One explanation is that people fear the reprisal that may be associated with 'blowing the whistle'.

The 2012 NHS staff survey provided an interesting insight into this issue. Although over 90 per cent of staff claimed to know how to raise concerns about poor or unsafe practice, only 72 per cent said that they would feel safe to do so. Even when nurses do know how to speak out about concerns the Royal College of Nursing suggest that just under half who responded to a survey stated that their employer took no action when they did so.

Thus the reasons why things go wrong are complex and multi-faceted but may be traceable back to the culture of the workplace. It is easy to suggest that there is a simple choice at work to speak out if things seem to be wrong – or to remain silent and get through the shift. However, workplace cultures are more complex than this and there are several other tactics that individuals employ to challenge the 'unwritten rules' that the sociologist Erving Goffman was so skilled at revealing in *Asylums* (1961).

I was involved in a research study with a colleague that explored different people's attitudes to whistleblowing in relation to the care of older people (Kelly and Jones, 2013). Included in the study were final-year undergraduate student nurses, as well as managers, home-care staff, the police and other healthcare professionals. The study focused on how these groups perceived whistleblowing and whether and when they might see themselves ever whistleblowing in their work with older people.

Some of their views are presented below, and in other parts of the chapter, and provide interesting insights into their perceptions of whistleblowing. When we asked managers who worked in older people's services what they thought about whistleblowing as a term they confirmed an overwhelmingly negative perception:

'I think it's kind of a negative effect isn't it with the wording of it, I think perhaps raising concern for individuals or something along those lines would be better. I think with a lot of the carers they feel as if they're sort of um, for want of a better word, grassing on their colleagues or say a family member or something if there's an issue with a service user.'

When this same question was put to third-year undergraduate nurses a range of views emerged:

Student nurse 1: 'People think it's a bad thing because it a called whistleblowing.'

Student Nurse 2: 'Yes.'

Student Nurse 1: 'It's like a grass or something.'

Student Nurse 3: 'It's a bit like being in the playground isn't it. If you are going to whistle-blow then you're going to tell on your friends and everybody wants to be popular at the end of the day they don't want to be seen as the one that's you know ...'

Student Nurse 4: 'Telling tales?'

Student Nurse 3: 'Yes, and stepping away from your peer group and what everyone else is doing, but obviously with something as serious as abuse or whatever it might be then you have to just put that to one side and do what you think is the right thing.'

In both examples it is possible to see the negative impact of going against one's colleagues and speaking out. Blowing the whistle is recognised by these individuals as a very risky choice of action that singles one out; but the students also could see times when it might be the only option.

These examples indicate that avoiding things going wrong cannot simply rely on 'good people doing the right thing' – although it certainly may eventually require that – but that it takes courage to be willing to make oneself speak out. This is why a sociological understanding of workplace cultures is relevant as you prepare for a career in nursing.

Without this perspective there is a risk of looking for overly simple solutions (such as relying upon or creating yet more whistleblowing policies) rather than asking 'What is the type of culture that exists here?', 'Are the patients cared for well and are the staff motivated and engaged in maintaining high standards?', 'Who has the power and how is this power used?' These questions might seem to be directed only towards those who are in positions of authority in the workplace, such as ward sisters/charge nurses, but the same, or very similar questions, will also apply to those who work more directly at the level of providing care on each shift to individual patients.

The impact of workplace culture on the operation of policies was a central finding from our whistleblowing research that you can read more about (Jones and Kelly, 2014b; Older Person's Commissioner for Wales, 2012). Workplace culture can be considered to arise from the general atmosphere, psychosocial climate or environment within which workers undertake their role. It determines the way people interact and can be understood as a unique combination of the behaviours, beliefs, morals and goals of which an organisation is comprised. We will now examine this issue in more depth and draw on an example from outside of healthcare and ask why some workplace cultures allow things to go wrong.

Workplace culture and the normalisation of deviance

The culture of the workplace has a strong bearing upon the worker's sense of values and commitment to the work; on their sense of achievement and ability to influence change; and even on their personal relationships and happiness. It can also determine what they value most about work and where their loyalties lie when problems arise.

Participants in our research into whistleblowing (Older Person's Commissioner for Wales, 2012), particularly managers, felt that a supportive workplace culture was vital to the raising of concerns. One spoke of the need to be aware of how the abnormal can soon become accepted as the norm in some workplaces:

'It's that sort of habituation of abnormal behaviours which then leads you to actually believe that, Oh it's okay, when in fact it's not. So there are some things which I believe people just accept which they shouldn't be doing, then it's up to us to police it as much as we can ... it even happens with the senses – because if you go to the floors, if people are working on those floors day in, day out, they don't smell if there's a scent of urine.

Yet I'll go there and I'll say 'I can smell urine can you please come and do something about this, it's obvious there's something in the carpet here or whatever,' and I mean that's a sensory thing, a sensory habituation, but there is a psychological habituation to it ...' (p. 11)

This echoes the research of Dianne Vaughan (1996) who highlights the gradual erosion of boundaries in the workplace regarding what is acceptable or safe, and what is not; gradually the unacceptable can become the norm.

Vaughan is a sociologist who examined the background to the launch of the *Challenger* space shuttle in 1986. The mission attracted much publicity as it included the first American schoolteacher, Christine McAuliffe, as part of the mission. Vaughan adopted a research method termed historical ethnography to systematically and critically explore the background to the launch and the culture at NASA at that time.

Her findings are intriguing as they reveal the way that everyday attitudes – what she terms 'institutional banalities' – allowed previously sacrosanct safety rules to be bent and eventually broken. This, in turn, led to the deviance she noted becoming institutionalised, resulting in 'an incremental descent into poor judgment'. It is not necessary to go into the technical details about the readiness of the shuttle to be launched here; however, the decision taken to launch on a particularly cold day in January 1986 resulted in disaster with all seven crew members losing their lives over the Atlantic Ocean.

Of note is Vaughan's description of decision-making the evening before when safety engineers warned against a launch due to abnormally low temperatures, but this was overruled due to decisions from people wearing a 'management hat'. By conducting the historical ethnography in this detailed way she revealed the fact that middle managers did not inform top management of previous safety conversations; a fact explained by the amount of financial and reputational risk at play.

In the end this research from the space industry can be seen to have close parallels with healthcare, which is also multi-layered and bureaucratised. In a culture driven by targets, or the need to cut costs, news of forthcoming disasters may be highly unwelcome. In such circumstances organisations may appear 'deaf' to warnings and the process of normalising deviance continues. This situation has been termed the 'deaf effect' (see below).

In our paper (Jones and Kelly, 2014a) you can read more about the concept of the deaf effect and why it occurs. This has been described as 'When a decision maker doesn't hear, ignores or overrules a report of bad news continue a failing course of action' (Cuellar, 2009: 23).

Previous research in health settings has also looked at workplace cultures and found that a 'closed, inward looking and insular' culture can lead to 'unprofessional, counter-therapeutic and degrading – even cruel – practices taking place' (Commission for Health Improvement, 2000: 10).

Vaughan's research also revealed co-existing cultures in NASA as a workplace; one she termed 'technical' which emphasised success and a 'can-do' attitude. The other, perhaps more dangerous, was a culture of 'secrecy' where problems were 'filtered' before being passed up the chain, leading to attention being paid to only one aspect of a task at the expense of all others.

Think here about the target culture of the NHS and the impact that waiting targets can have further along the line when beds are required and people may be discharged before they are ready, or routine procedures may be cancelled again and again due to lack of beds. Can you see similarities with the findings from NASA in the 1980s?

Scenario 7.1   Notes on a scandal

The final report into unnecessary deaths, poor care, understaffing and inaction against concerns at Mid Staffordshire NHS Foundation Trust was published in 2013 (a weblink has been provided at the end of this chapter if you wish to access this report). However, it is clear that concerns had been raised much earlier – certainly since 2005. In fact there were 940 concerns recorded as having been submitted to the National Patient Safety Agency. As well as formal written concerns there was evidence of an avoidance of responsibility and a culture of 'not bringing bad news to the boardroom'. The Director of Nursing at the time later claimed that her title was misleading as nursing management was actually 'delegated'.

A junior doctor working in A&E had complained to the trust board and then to the medical deanery who took no action regarding his concerns. He said that the emergency department in the hospital routinely resembled a disaster area and those working there appeared 'immune to the sound of pain'.

Refer back to the scenario that opened this chapter about the lady being found in a state of distress and undress and it is possible to see evidence of the closed, inward looking and insular culture described above.

The human suffering that was unearthed in this situation at Mid Staffordshire culminated in the finding that an elevated mortality rate was also evident. During the inquiry experts were asked to comment on whether the higher mortality rate was due to data-quality problems, or to bad care. Arguments on both sides were offered. However, whether we accept the explanations given or not we can once again see the symptoms of a workplace culture that had closed in on itself in an attempt try to explain why things went so badly wrong. Sir Robert Francis, who chaired the inquiry, said: 'Let us all hope that in the near future we will stop having to listen to disturbing reports of poor and unsafe care.'

When you read about the scandal at Mid Staffs, and there have been many others over the years, you may wonder why this can be allowed to happen. Clearly concerns were raised through 'official channels' but still no one seemed to take action. The culture that had grown up around this hospital was such that employees may have felt powerless to act, even if they had information or personal experience to hand. Do you feel confident that the hope expressed by Robert Francis will be realised or do you have doubts? If there are doubts can we use our sociological insights into organisations, and how they function, to help prevent such situations? Does the work of Dianne Vaughan into the *Challenger* disaster have resonances in Mid Staffordshire?

At the heart of the issue of poor or unsafe care is not only the workplace culture but also the individual practitioners, including student or registered nurses, who work within systems that exist to support vulnerable people. Vulnerability is itself a broad concept and can include people in emergency situations as well as those living for many years with dementia, learning difficulties or chronic physical or mental health conditions.

The numbers of people diagnosed with dementia alone is rising at an unprecedented rate so it is important to be aware of the challenge we are going to face as individuals, and as a society, to provide cultures of care that are humane and person-centred; rather than settings that risk 'going wrong'. The demand on primary and secondary care is unlikely to diminish as estimates suggest that by 2025 the number of people living with dementia alone is expected to rise to over one million and by 2050 it is projected to exceed two million (Lewis et al., 2014)

As has been discussed in the other chapters throughout this book, nursing work involves a complex mix of skills, attitudes, emotional labour and managing the expectations placed on nurses to provide an appropriate caring response regardless of the demands placed upon them. This is not easy work, and we do not underestimate the commitment it takes to provide good care; often with insufficient staff, lack of resources and rarely with enough time.

To help us in our thinking about why and how things can go wrong it would be useful at this point to build further upon Dianne Vaughan's work and consider some other important sociological research into institutions described as 'closed' in some way to the outside world. Some of the most influential research in this field was carried out in large psychiatric hospitals or units where patients (and staff) had been present for many years. Erving Goffman in his classic study *Asylums* (1961) referred to such places as 'total institutions', referring to the extreme forms of socialisation processes that shaped every aspect of life, and permeated all layers of function, in these places.

Taken in context this work by Erving Goffman is characteristic of sociological research of the early 1960s – often described as a time of dissent in medical sociology; when critiques of the dominant structural-functionalism (see Chapter 1) led to new – and highly significant – studies that still have relevance today (Collyer, 2012).

Goffman's *Asylums* had broken away from the dominance of structural-functionalism that offered a general theory of society but also led to one of the most influential theories in medical sociology – that of the 'sick role' by Talcott Parsons in 1951 (see Chapters 1 and 2).

Goffman had championed the importance of researching and recording everyday life and relishing what can usefully be revealed by 'ethnographies of the self'. He and his research have since been much praised, exemplified in this warm tribute by another sociologist Elliot Freidson in 1983:

> First, Goffman's early work is focused on the individual self, in a world that at once creates and oppresses it. Second, Goffman's work is intensely moral in character, marked by a passionate defense of the self against society. And third, Goffman's work has no systematic relationship to abstract academic theory and provides no encouragement to attempt to advance such theory. What gives Goffman's work a value that will endure far longer than most sociology is its intense individual humanity and its style. (p. 359)

Asylums is often cited as leading to the de-institutionalisation of many long-stay mental health hospitals and the book can still captivate the reader with rich descriptions of institutional life, even after so many years.

You may want to try reading sections of *Asylums* or *The Presentation of Self in Everyday Life* (see Chapter 5) and see if they resonate with your experiences in placements. You might want to compare what you are learning in practice about being 'a professional self' with what you learn in your academic studies.

The importance of Goffman's contribution was also illustrated in a special edition of the *British Journal of Psychiatry* in 2011. The editorial (Mac Suibhne, 2011) summarised Goffman's role in helping to humanise psychiatric care in general:

> Erving Goffman's *Asylums: Essays on the Social Situation of Mental Patients and Other Inmates* is a key text in the sociology of mental illness. It is sometimes seen simplistically as a paradigm of 'antipsychiatry', and as a key step in the triumph of community psychiatry over narrower, medical models of mental illness. Reading *Asylums* today, however, reveals that this portrayal does not capture the richness of the text. My argument is that, rather than being an opponent of biological psychiatry or medical models *per se*, Goffman's key role was in humanising patients and drawing attention to the patterns of interaction that dehumanised them.

In relation to the quote that opened this chapter by the daughter of the patient covered in faeces, Goffman's work *The Presentation of Self in Everyday Life* (1959) can also provide insight into the reasons why this situation is so shocking from a sociological, as well as a moral, perspective:

> In our society, defecation involves an individual in activity which is defined as inconsistent with the cleanliness and purity standards expressed in many of our performances. Such activity also causes the individual to disarrange his clothing and to 'go out of play', that is, to drop from his face the expressive mask that he employs in face-to-face interaction. At the same time it becomes difficult for him to reassemble his personal front should the need to enter into interaction suddenly occur. Perhaps that is a reason why toilet doors in our society have locks on them. (p. 121)

Thus it is possible to see a connection between Goffman's theorising about human toilet behaviour – and the strong social boundaries that govern this normally private body function – and the shock of witnessing a loved one in such a state in Mid Staffordshire NHS Trust. The culture of this workplace can be seen to have deviated so much from the norm that this patient's situation and distress was deemed acceptable (or at least was not considered a priority).

Goffman's work also reminds us that social rules that underpin the culture of total institutions are not written down (at least not in the depth to which they shaped every aspect of the culture) but they are extremely pervasive and powerful. To survive in such settings patients and staff had to learn quickly about what was acceptable and what was not. Going against the tide of such powerful social practices took courage as one must reject the dominant culture, and accept the risks involved to one's future career.

Whistleblowing and its alternatives

Reflection 7.2

Think about your first day on a recent placement. This could be somewhere that you had never worked before. You will hopefully have been met by a mentor or other colleague and introduced to 'the routine' of your new workplace and how things are done here. Try to remember how it felt to be a stranger in this new setting. What was your very first impression? If you were asked to give a word to describe this place what would it be? What were the sights and smells; what noise did you hear? Did you get any impressions about the people working there and if they seemed happy? Think about how you tried to 'read' these people and to fit in. Think about the person in charge and their style of leadership. Did they talk to you and if so was that helpful? What is the attitude of the team to this workplace and to the work itself? What are the helpful things you need to feel more comfortable and to fit in? Did you think people were proud of their work? Did you feel the care was of a good standard?

Keep these first impressions in mind and think about whether they changed over time as you started to 'fit in'.

As you undertake your undergraduate education, and then qualify as a registered nurse, you may come across situations in clinical practice that you feel concerned about. The attitudes of the staff you are working with may be worrying – they may be competent but seem less than kind in their attitudes to patients; or you may feel that the routines that you are expected to work to seem to be more beneficial to the staff themselves than to the patients.

Very occasionally you may feel so concerned about the standard of care or what you see happening that you feel you have to act and report it.

As well as hospital events these situations can also arise in a person's home where they may be socially isolated and reliant on nurses or care workers as their only source of social contact. In these cases you may find that there is limited time to spend with each patient due to caseload numbers. This can feel frustrating as you may be able to provide what may be considered adequate levels of care; but it may not reach the standard that you believe these patients really need.

When considering such situations we may consider them 'micro' in nature, in that they are impacting on individuals (patients and nurses) rather than being about the NHS more widely. However, they are the result of 'macro' societal-level questions about how we fund, design and deliver healthcare needs for vulnerable people (Machell et al., 2009). We should be concerned by recent reports into care that is sometimes far from satisfactory for older patients in hospital settings who may not receive help with the most basic of needs such as having enough food, fluids and skin care. The dignity of such patients is also compromised, which implies that a culture of neglect (once again via the normalisation of deviance) may be worryingly pervasive.

You can find an example of such concerns here from a recent study carried out in English hospitals: www.theguardian.com/society/2015/jul/15/nhs-care-of-elderly-patients-often-poor-and-lacking-dignity-report-says.

Examples from this study revealed examples of patients who were not treated with dignity and respect and the numbers who were not helped to eat in the 'vast majority' of NHS hospitals was high.

The researcher found that almost a quarter of patients reported having experienced poor or inconsistent standards of dignity and respect. One in three who needed help eating did not receive it. When all older people were considered, women, those aged over 80 years and those with a chronic illness or disability, such as blindness or deafness, were most at risk of receiving care that was inadequate.

What these findings suggest is that problems exist for the most vulnerable patients and there is a need to act on concerns before they deteriorate to an extent that standards may be difficult to recover.

This situation has similarities with the work of Barry Turner in the late 1970s who proposed the 'man-made disaster' theory. In this he suggested the gradual disruption to what he called 'human and socio-technical systems' to manage complex risks or problems (Turner, 1978). This may be despite the best of intentions to prevent such events but failure occurs due to gradual and significant disruption to cultural beliefs and accepted norms about safety, hazards and standards. Pidgeon and O'Leary (2000) discuss this further and argue:

> All organisations operate within such cultural beliefs and norms, which might be formally laid down in rules and procedures, or more tacitly taken for granted and embedded within working practices ... there are always very many pre-conditions to any major systems failure, some originating years prior to the actual event. (p. 16)

Turner (1978) terms this time lag the 'incubation period' which is especially relevant in terms of the focus of this chapter as things rarely go wrong suddenly. Instead it may take many years for the situation to gradually build in a workplace that shows features of being 'closed' to concerns that are raised by staff or relatives. Once again we can see connections with the work of Erving Goffman on the power of the total institution and Dianne Vaughan's theory of the normalisation of deviance.

In healthcare the importance of delay or the 'incubation of concerns' can be seen in the way that incidents, or other sources of feedback such as complaints, are listened to and dealt with (or, alternatively, ignored) (Kelly and Jones 2013, Jones and Kelly, 2014a). The apparently simple choice of speaking out or staying silent, however, is not so clear when organisations fail to respond to concerns, even when there is a build-up of events to the point when disaster occurs.

The managers and student nurses in our study into whistleblowing reinforced the need to listen to staff as this is the first stage in any process to manage concerns about standards of care:

> 'To me it really doesn't matter, the important thing whatever you call it is if people have concerns to say so, which I hope that we do here. It's academic what it's called isn't it really? ... And I think if people are told that it's okay to come and speak up then I don't think it should bother them what it's called, as long as they're told that it's okay there won't be repercussions you know, they need to know that so whatever you call it.' (Manager)

'I think that's a positive thing because of that, because I mean it's good to be able to call someone for help, it's like whistling for help, for someone from outside to come in and help you if there is no one inside the ward is willing to resolve the issue. So I can see that as a positive thing. I mean, it sounds a bit scary but ...' (Student nurse)

There was also agreement that whistleblowing represented a serious step; and one that they might only consider if events were considered significantly 'major' or 'serious'. This is exemplified below in two extracts from a focus group with student nurses:

Q. 'What comes to your head when you think of whistleblowing? Do you think it's a positive term or not?'

'No. It kind of something really bad has happened, doesn't it, it's not just like little things in practice that need to ... it's something dramatic that every ... It's fundamental like ... Yes.'

'When I think of whistleblowing I think of really serious things like that nurse Beverley Allitt or when patients are badly abused. The sort of really serious things you see on the television or read in a newspaper.'

Importantly, and in terms of how subtle features of workplace culture can be used to effect change, the study also revealed how humour could sometimes be used as an informal means of informing colleagues about concerns. This could include the way care is being delivered – such as the way a patient with dementia is being fed. The following quote is an example of this from a healthcare assistant working in a care home:

'Sometimes I need to say something but, instead of going for it, I'd try and draw attention by laughing and saying something like, 'Oh, she's in a rush 'cos she's going out tonight' or something, you know, if they were feeding a patient too quickly or taking a plate away without giving them a proper chance to finish. Sometimes you get a look and you know it has hit home.'

The 'look' referred to in this quote is a simple yet powerful social gesture that acted as a corrective signal in this workplace. When care tasks, such as feeding or toileting, become so everyday and routinised then the policing function by this healthcare assistant could be viewed as an important intervention – and one that had some effect; but it did not need to be escalated to the point of speaking to a manager, or referring to a written concerns policy.

Instead the informal mechanism of making it known that something about this co-worker's behaviour was less than acceptable by commenting in a light-hearted way reveals an example of challenging the social rules. These rules will include task completion and time management that will govern the structured work of these teams. The support worker's choice of action can be seen as significant (but it may also carry the risk of being seen as critical, untrustworthy, or not one of the team if done too often).

In this sense social interaction within this care home has revealed at least some features of the 'total institution' described by Goffman (1961). By this he meant that people shared a similar social situation (washing, dressing, feeding and interacting with the same colleagues each day). In care-home settings staff routinely work closely with vulnerable and highly dependent older people, some of whom may have severe cognitive deficits, and who may be unable to interact appropriately with their care givers (refusing care aggressively for example).

Those working in such settings can also be seen as being separated from the norms of wider society for several hours each day. This can result in a 'formally administered round of life' as Goffman described it in *Asylums* (1961: 11), meaning that anyone who speaks out against this round of life – even informally – risks standing out and being considered untrustworthy. Thus the act of correction described by this young care assistant above should not be underestimated – she had raised her concerns but in a way that both saved face with her co-workers (see Chapter 5) and prevented her having to side with authority figures. A formal whistleblowing approach would have required the opposite approach, which is why some of the nurses who spoke in our whistleblowing study considered this alternative 'scary':

> 'Well it sounds, I don't like the word, because it sounds as though you are doing some-thing bad you know. It's like you are grassing on people whereas you're not really, you're raising a concern aren't you and you want to make someone aware of the situ-ation. The whistleblowing thing sounds awful to me like you're doing something devious and sneaky and behind somebody's back and I'm sure they could find a better word than that ...'

These sentiments should perhaps be recalled when whistleblowing policies for use in the workplace are being created. Other terms have recently been promoted such as 'speaking up' or 'raising concerns'; however, the sociological importance attached to workplace culture, and the features that govern people's everyday behaviour within institutions, have a clear relevance for understanding why some things can and do go wrong. Importantly we do not need to work in 'total institutions', as Goffman described them, for this issue to be relevant.

There are also alternatives to consider in terms of preventing concerns becoming so significant that whistleblowing might be required. Strategies have been intro-duced to encourage healthcare students to think about the care they are providing and to improve it in small, incremental steps each day, or each time they interact with a patient (Carson-Stevens et al., 2013). This is a simple yet powerful approach to everyday interactions that acknowledges the vulnerability of the patient and helps prevent the creep of institutional thinking. The simple act of asking someone 'What one thing can I do to improve your care today?' could range from something as simple as 'please give me some ice in my water jug' to 'please explain why I'm taking these tablets'.

Asking colleagues the same question 'What one thing would improve your working life?' is another way to ensure that organisations can be seen to listen and respond on an ongoing basis to their staff. The same question can also be asked at the level of care delivery as well as across managerial/institutional boundaries where differ-ent people may require different things to improve their working life – by doing so we might hear concerns in a more honest and speedy way without having recourse to whistleblowing at all.

When things go wrong in other ways: avoidant leadership and bullying

Whether concerns are raised formally or informally the outcome will always be unpredictable. Indeed there is a growing body of research that shows that some authority figures, including nurse managers, may not act as expected in such situations. In Chapter 8 you can read more about leadership and management theory and some of the sociological insights that have informed our understanding of its function in healthcare systems.

However, some of these theories of leadership or management may appear rather idealistic; especially in the context of considering what happens when things are going wrong. Jackson et al. (2012) have contributed a useful understanding of an additional range of leadership behaviours that also may be relevant; these are negative and considered 'avoidant' in nature. By this is meant leaders who display three possible responses when concerns are raised:

- The first is termed 'placatory' where leaders may affirm staff concerns but then fail to act.
- The second type of avoidant response is termed 'equivocal' and describes the leader appearing ambivalent about the concern being raised and also failing to act.
- The final type is described as 'hostile' and is where the leader reacts to the person who raises the concern in a manner that causes feelings of hostility to be experienced. They may also fail to act.

These insights have relevance to the overall message of this chapter where it has been argued that the culture of the workplace is key in shaping people's (including your own) behaviour. Inevitably people will only raise concerns, either informally or formally, if they believe that leaders will be receptive to them. If they do not feel confident about this then the risks associated with closed workplace cultures, where concerns are hidden away and not passed upwards and acted upon, can lead to disasters such as was seen at Mid Staffs NHS Foundation Trust, or at NASA 30 years ago.

This is also relevant as those who do report concerns place themselves in a vulnerable position. Whilst they may not consider themselves whistleblowers (with all the associated negative connotations discussed earlier) they will have exposed their opinions enough to challenge the dominant culture that may usually involve silence, secrecy (and sometimes shame) in some 'closed' workplaces. This is made worse if leaders then fail to act despite the individual taking the risk of speaking out.

However, it is also true that leaders may be more open and responsive, and those in authority may seek to transform a problematic situation into a much more positive one. A recent study by myself and colleagues (Kelly et al., 2015) invited executive nurse directors in England and Wales to speak about their roles and the impact of the findings of the Francis Report (2013). The respondents emphasised ongoing challenges such as workload demands, political and financial pressures on NHS trusts and health boards, the need for supportive colleagues at board level and (sometimes) poor collegial relationships in senior teams. More acute challenges were described as dealing with complaints or concerns about sub-optimal standards of care or responding to crises, such as outbreaks of infections.

These insights into the reality of senior nursing roles are helpful in demonstrating that workload pressures exist at all levels in health systems, and the way that individuals respond throughout is shaped by personal approaches to the role and the culture in which they work. Some executive nurse directors were able to manage the pressures by developing ways of relaxing and managing time pressures – the same skills of resilience that were presented for consideration by yourself and clinical colleagues at the end of Chapter 5.

It is also important to maintain some healthy scepticism, as the external image portrayed by an organisation – such as an NHS trust – may be very different to what happens in the reality of clinical settings. The idealised version that exists may be threatened by the nature of the concern being raised, such as uncaring staff (see Chapter 5 for an example of a job advertisement for a fictitious workplace that espouses very high values about everyone who works there). Thus organisational reputations can be put at risk by those who do choose to report concerns. Different responses may be expected to preserve the unit or an organisation's reputation by trying to stop the person speaking out. Negative responses may include ignoring (by avoidant leadership described earlier) by scapegoating or through bullying behaviours by colleagues and/or managers.

When the response to colleagues is characteristic of bullying this may be because those with responsibility fear they will be made to lose face (again see Chapter 5) or will be judged to have been complicit in condoning poor or unsafe practices. This can result in retaliation against the individual in the form of alienation from the peer group or more overt bullying.

Bullying in nursing has been a topic researched for some time by colleagues with an interest in workplace behaviour. Studies have used exploratory research methods to describe bullying situations that nurses may find themselves in. For examples of research into bullying in nursing see the work of Hutchinson et al. (2006, 2010). Leaders who display avoidant responses to concerns may also fail to respond to reports of bullying behaviour, so further undermining the ethical climate of the workplace.

Reflection 7.3

In a recent article in the (Hazell, 2015) one NHS trust's bullying policy was considered not 'fit for purpose'. Do you have any experience of bullying in the workplace and if so can you describe what happened and how was it dealt with (if at all)? How was the bullying behaviour demonstrated? Can you think of reasons why the bullying was taking place and the extent to which it shaped the workplace culture? Have you ever seen bullying if someone you worked with raised concerns about the quality of patient care? Thinking about it now can you think of ways that this situation could have been managed differently?

Speaking truth to power, and to yourself

Finding a way to speak up when things go wrong is not easy and this chapter cannot offer quick solutions. However, by thinking in a sociological way about this topic you may come to a different way of understanding the power of workplace cultures and why things can go so badly wrong. If you further look into the literature on this topic you will see that more attention is being placed on raising concerns in healthcare than ever before. The references at the end of this chapter will give you the opportunity to explore this literature further.

In the whistleblowing study we discussed earlier there were some findings to feel more optimistic about and it was apparent that avoidant leadership was not a common trait. Indeed some managers were attempting to develop 'open-door' strategies to ensure that staff could access them and tell them how things really were.

Some examples include the two managers quoted below, one from a community homecare service and one in a care home for older people, who said:

'Quite frankly, I'm one of these people "better out than in", you know? And I'd rather that we opened things up and looked and healed and dealt with things.'

'I'm trying to be a positive role model in this, you know, I say the door's open, come and see me but when I was a junior staff nurse I was never encouraged to do that ...'

As well as more positive attitudes such as these it is also important to note that those in power (including managers, NHS boards, politicians and regulatory bodies) are acutely aware that poor care and the mistreatment of patients is always 'bad news'. The reputational risk involved in admitting to failure, therefore, is itself likely to remain a significant barrier to prevent workplace cultures being completely open. Perhaps this will never be completely possible due to the need for confidentiality and privacy in healthcare services. To this end the advice to anyone seeking to 'speak truth to power' is to gather as much evidence as possible and to seek help and advice in the process.

There are sources of information readily available, such as the Royal College of Nursing (RCN) website. The message behind recent campaigns to invite nurses to report resource shortages is included in the box below. The Frontline First took place in 2014/15 is an example only. The RCN launch new campaigns regularly in response to changing circumstances and the most up to date information can be found on the RCN website www.rcn.org.uk

Reflection 7.4   Cuts to jobs and services

The NHS is facing one of the most challenging periods in its 60-year history as the government looks to find billions of pounds of efficiency savings.

Across the UK, individual NHS organisations continue to announce plans for efficiency savings which are likely to impact on services and jobs. You are in a position to see first-hand the cuts that are being made in your local area.

Concluding remarks

The closing message of this chapter is to encourage you to be aware of the insights that sociological theory can provide to help you to understand the culture in which you work. When you feel things are going wrong there are ways to consider the options available and to reach a resolution that feels right for you. This need not necessarily involve a large-scale scandal where care is so poor that you feel lives are at stake (but of course this could be the case). Instead it could be that you feel uncomfortable with the attitudes and approach of your co-workers towards patients. Care may be provided on the surface but it feels as if it is lacking in humanity or connection with the suffering of the individuals involved.

In such cases you might find it useful to think about some of the insights provided in this book on the role of nursing; power differentials between different professions; the status of those who provide nursing care; and the nature of workplace cultures that combine to create a situation that you feel uncomfortable with.

At these times you will now be able to develop an understanding of why such situations arise by considering the work of sociologists, such as Goffman and Vaughan, who have provided us with insights into 'total institutions', 'closed cultures' and the 'normalisation of deviance'.

Remember that concerns about care standards can exist on different scales and can range from poor performance of an entire NHS trust down to individual wards or units, or indeed certain teams or individuals working on a particular rota.

With these insights there remain questions for you to consider in your role as a nurse, and for all nurses who may find themselves witnesses of poor care, and who fail to act or report it; as well as other members of the healthcare team who also fail to respond in the face of wrongdoing or unacceptable standards. In the end this a personal decision and personal morality is the best guide available.

Chapter summary

In a sociological sense this chapter has shown that things go wrong because we are all 'social actors' and we each play a role – part of this role is developing our own sense of agency and choice and to do something that might prevent a potentially bad situation becoming worse. The chapter has introduced you to some key theories and examples of recent events, as well as research studies that you may want to read more about.

However, the chapter also ends with a word of caution – if we are all playing a part in healthcare then we are all culpable in some way when things go wrong; and we are all at risk as future recipients of healthcare services as a result.

The resistance that, as individuals, we can choose to show will mean we may sometimes have to go against powerful workplace cultures that are promoting at best mediocre, and at worst dangerous, care. The choice about what to do is always personal but the gain involved in speaking truth to power can be summed up in the words of Erving Goffman:

> It is ... *against something* that the self can emerge ... Our sense of being a person can come from being drawn into a wider social unit; our sense of selfhood can arise through the little ways in which we resist the pull. (1961: 320)

Going further

RCN resource on dealing with bullying and harassment: www2.rcn.org.uk/__data/assets/pdf_file/0011/78518/001497.pdf.

A relevant article on the total institution: Goodman, B. (2012) Erving Goffman and the total institution. *Nurse Education Today* 33: 81–82.

National Archives weblink for the final Report on the Inquiry into the Mid Staffordshire NHS Foundation Trust: http://webarchive.nationalarchives.gov.uk/20150407084003/www.midstaffspublicinquiry.com/.

References

Carson-Stevens, A., Jones, A., Hansen, A.S., Printz, A., Patel, E., Bhatt, J. and Panesar, S.S. (2013) 'What can I do to improve your care today?' One question closer to patient-centered care. *American Journal of Medical Quality* 28: 174.

Collyer, F. (2012) *Mapping the Sociology of Health and Medicine*. Basingstoke: Palgrave.

Commission for Health Improvement (2000) *Inquiry Report into the North Lakeland Trust: Report to the Secretary of State for Health*. London.

Cuellar, M. (2009) An investigation of the deaf effect response to bad news reporting in information systems projects. Unpublished PhD thesis, Georgia State University.

Francis, R. (2013) *Report on the Mid Staffordshire NHS Foundation Trust Public Inquiry*. London: The Stationery Office.

Freidson, E. (1983) Celebrating Erving Goffman. *Contemporary Sociology* 12(4): 359–362.

Goffman, E. (1959) *The Presentation of Self in Everyday Life*. New York: Doubleday.

Goffman, E. (1961) *Asylums*. New York: Doubleday & Anchor.

Hazell, W. (2015) Worcestershire trust's bullying policy 'not fit for purpose'. *Health Service Journal*, 27 August.

Hutchinson, M., Vickers, M., Jackson, D. and Wilkes, L. (2006) Like wolves in a pack: predatory alliances of bullies in nursing. *Journal of Management and Organisation* 12: 235–250.

Hutchinson, M., Vickers, M., Jackson, D. and Wilkes, L (2010) Bullying as circuits of power: an Australian nursing perspective. *Administrative Theory and Praxis* 3: 25–47.

Jackson, D., Hutchinson, M., Peters, K. and Luck, L. (2012) Understanding avoidant leadership in healthcare: findings from a secondary analysis of two qualitative studies. *Journal of Nursing Management* 21: 572–580.

Jones, A. and Kelly, D. (2014a) Deafening silence? Time to reconsider whether organisations are silent or deaf when things go wrong. *BMJ Quality & Safety* 23: 709–713.

Jones, A. and Kelly, D. (2014b) Whistleblowing and workplace culture in older people's care: qualitative insights from the healthcare and social care workforce. *Sociology of Health & Illness* 36: 986–1002.

Kelly, D.M. and Jones, A. (2013) When care is needed: The role of whistleblowing in promoting best standards from an individual and organizational perspective. *Quality in Ageing and Older Adults* 14(3): 180–191.

Kelly, D., Lankshear, A. and Jones, A. (2015) *Resilient Leadership in a Time of Crisis: Experiences of Executive Directors of Nursing in the Wake of the Francis Report*. Report to the GNC Trust. Cardiff: Cardiff University.

Lewis, F., Schaffer, S., Sussex, J., O'Neil, P. and Cockcroft, L. (2014) *The Trajectory of Dementia in the UK – Making a Difference*. London: Alzheimer's Research UK and the Office of Health Economics.

Mac Suibhne, S. (2011) Erving Goffman's *Asylum* fifty years on. *British Journal of Psychiatry* 198: 1–2.

Machell, S., Gough, P. and Steward, K. (2009) *From Ward to Board: Identifying Good Practice in the Business of Caring*. London: The King's Fund.

Older Person's Commissioner for Wales (2012) Raising concerns in the workplace. Final report. Available at www.olderpeoplewales.com.

Parsons, T. (1951) *The Social System*. London: Routledge & Kegan Paul.

Pidgeon, N. and O'Leary, M. (2000) Man-made disasters: why technology and organizations (sometimes) fail. *Safety Science* 34: 15–30.

Turner, B. (1978) *Man-Made Disasters*. London: Butterworth-Heinemann.

Vaughan, D. (1996) *The Challenger Launch Decision: Risky Technology, Culture, and Deviance at NASA*. Chicago: University of Chicago Press.

8

Leadership and management

Michael Traynor

Issue

In this chapter we consider how sociological theory can help us understand issues related to leadership and management in nursing, midwifery and the National Health Service (NHS) more broadly.

Consider the following extracts from the Report of the Mid Staffordshire NHS Foundation Trust Public Inquiry (Francis, 2013):

> It has not escaped the Inquiry's notice that even since the HCC [Healthcare Commission] report on the [Mid Staffordshire] Trust there have been a series of highly concerning reports of experiences elsewhere containing echoes of what was experienced within the Trust ... Even if all the instances contained in the reports just mentioned are in some way isolated ones dependant on particular circumstances, they are suggestive that there are places where unhealthy cultures, poor leadership, and an acceptance of poor standards are too prevalent. (p. 25)

> As a result of poor leadership and staffing policies, a completely inadequate standard of nursing was offered on some wards in Stafford. The complaints heard at both the first inquiry and this one testified not only to inadequate staffing levels, but poor leadership, recruitment and training. This led in turn to a declining professionalism and a tolerance of poor standards. (p. 45)

It is a truism that organisational culture is informed by the nature of its leadership. (p. 64)

The common culture and values of the NHS must be applied at all levels of the organisation, but of particular importance is the example set by leaders. (p. 78)

Look at a report into any recent scandal in the NHS and you are likely find at least part of the blame apportioned to a 'lack of leadership'. 'Leadership' at least for the last 35 years has been seen as the solution to a global range of problems and challenges, from international economic competitiveness to the need to motivate staff in an NHS hospital ward. But some of this faith in leadership is based on assumptions and myths, fuelled by a multi-billion dollar industry involving leadership and management institutes, training courses and paperback publications, as well as media promotions of stereotypes of business and media managers. In this chapter, as with every chapter in this book, we want to question this powerful set of taken-for-granted assumptions and explore where these ideas came from, in what social and economic contexts and where their inconsistencies and problems might lie. Of course ideas about leadership and good management do have usefulness – once we get past the exaggerated expectations and the poorly thought-through assumptions. Groups of people can work together either relatively well or extremely poorly and some of this is down to how those in charge conduct themselves. Recent reports about patient safety (Berwick, 2013) and poorly performing NHS trusts (Keogh, 2013) give some practical guidance about effective leadership. The work of organisational psychologists also reveals the usefulness of good approaches to leadership (West, 2014).

We will start our exploration by considering ideas about leadership in general and then focus on leadership as it is talked about within the UK health service and in the nursing profession, and how these two are different and potentially in tension. Many commentators have asked the question whether leadership differs from 'management' and most conclude that leadership is a rather more exciting pastime. We will also be looking at this question. Finally, we discuss the often-neglected topic of how nurses delegate work to and manage healthcare support workers.

Chapter outline

In this chapter we will introduce and discuss the following sociological concepts:

- Bureaucracy and leadership
- The origins of the leadership industry
- Styles and forms of leadership
- Leadership in healthcare and managerialism
- Women and NHS leadership
- Professional leadership in nursing
- Delegation in healthcare and the division of labour

Bureaucracy and leadership

To start to look at leadership let's look at something different and perhaps contrasting first, a way of organising work in large organisations that has come to be known as bureaucracy. Once we have an understanding of the spirit of bureaucracy it will help us to appreciate just how different leadership can be, or at least how it has been conceived. The word bureaucracy is a mixture of French, *bureau* meaning desk or office, and the Greek κράτος *kratos*, meaning rule or political power, and when first used referred to government administrations that today we would understand as the civil service. We could apply it today to any large NHS organisation. Bureaucracy has key features, most of which we take for granted nowadays within the world of work:

- There is an emphasis on the office; that is, the role itself and not the individual who fulfils it. The work can pass from one post holder to another if the first were to leave.
- Unlike work in the Middle Ages, the bureaucratic office separates official activity from the sphere of private life.
- The management of the organisation follows general stable rules and office holders need to undertake technical learning to be able to follow these rules.
- The office holder in a bureaucracy is not expected to profit personally from the work but to hold office and fulfil it faithfully in return for a secure existence.
- Loyalty in a bureaucracy is not to a person but to the office itself, to a functional purpose rather than an individual.

Max Weber, who wrote extensively about bureaucracies and from whose work the above summary is taken, conceived of the professional bureaucrat as efficient and necessary to the functioning of modern society, but he also deplored the idea of the creature of petty routine lacking in heroism, spontaneity and inventiveness (Gerth and Wright Mills, 1997). Against this model of bureaucratic activity he set 'charismatic' leadership. The charismatic leader, for him, was a self-appointed individual who was followed by those in distress or who were convinced by his (and examples tended to be male) extraordinary qualities. Such leaders were revolutionary figures in history. Today's call for leadership in the NHS or in the professions is a call, as we understand it, for individuals to stand out against bureaucratic rationality, such as an NHS organisation that has developed highly systematised ways of controlling costs but needs to be recalled to its humanistic duty. The charismatic leader is not someone who has acquired expert knowledge like the bureaucrat, but someone considered to have a unique gift (the term means 'gift of grace') to which most have no access. The founders of religions are usually given as examples of this kind of leader, although we often only have very simple records written by their devotees of how they actually led so it is easy to be looking at highly idealised accounts. Today an overused list of a handful of recent generally popular and usually male political leaders, such as Martin Luther King, Gandhi and Winston Churchill, supplements this inventory.[1]

---

[1]Weber, however, claimed that a study of history shows that charismatic leadership is unstable and that the followers of charismatic leaders end up having to set up formal practices and institutes in order to maintain and extend the ideals of the leader. See Chapter 1 for further details about Weber.

But perhaps these kinds of emotive calls to consider examples of human greatness are a distraction and we need to look at the recent origins of the focus on leadership to understand more clearly how it affects us today.

Origins of leadership training

Today's discussion of management and leadership can be traced to the rise of business schools in the US and Europe and this is in turn linked to the intensification of industrial production and the increasing complexity of civil administration that were seen in the late nineteenth and early twentieth centuries in those regions. The first business schools were founded in Europe and the first in the UK was created in 1902 in Birmingham. In the US, the first business school was the Wharton School at the University of Pennsylvania. It was funded by a wealthy industrialist Joseph Wharton who was concerned that the country's current apprenticeship system would not deliver enough capable leaders in a period of rapid industrialisation. The School was associated with an influential group of businessmen, bankers and lawyers. Shortly after, in 1908, Harvard Business School was founded with a mission to train young people for a career in business, in the same way that medical school trained people for a career in medicine. It was the first business school to offer the now well-known MBA (Masters in Business Administration) programme. It has a stellar list of alumni, receives significant donations from successful business leaders and has a style and standard that other business schools aspire to. Many business schools are associated with high prestige corporations and conspicuous achievement. With notable exceptions the identification of business schools with entrepreneurial and financial success has marginalised critical or radical enquiry into management, management practices and leadership – by which we mean asking sometimes uncomfortable questions about its purpose and effects. However, the work of individuals at Lund University in Sweden and at the universities of Essex and Leicester in the UK, for example, has challenged many of the assumptions that conventional work in business and management accepts. These assumptions centre on the belief that the manager's role is to maximise production. A growing field of work, Critical Management Studies, looks at the unintended consequences of the promotion of management and leadership and draws on and makes significant contributions to social science theories of work, organisation and leadership, and we will discuss some of this work later in this chapter.

In addition to the work of academic business schools, the West has seen a growth in popular books, organisations and Internet sites promoting particular ideas about business success, often closely identified with a charismatic and successful individual. The 1980s saw the landmark book *In Search of Excellence: Lessons from America's Best-Run Companies* by Tom Peters and Robert H. Waterman and subsequently Peters has produced a large number of books. Peters' website describes him as 'almost single-handedly "inventing" the public "management guru industry," now global in scope and billions of dollars in size' (http://tompeters.com/about/toms-bio/). Note the strong element of individual heroism, an almost essential feature of such popular presentations of leadership. Even though the leader in question may be presenting a more nuanced version of leadership, it is their own successes that are drawn on to give them the authority to tell others how to do it. The stereotype of the charismatic business leader continues to fascinate and is promoted widely on television in programmes such as the BBC's *The Apprentice*. The enjoyment is in watching the business leader, in this series Alan Sugar, wield decisive personal power. So despite evidence to the contrary and more up-to-date ideas in organisational studies, leadership is still strongly influenced by individualistic ideas.

Styles and forms of leadership

Styles and forms of leadership were discussed in antiquity but the more recent manifestation probably originates from the early decades of the twentieth century. These styles are often presented as a taxonomy of contrasting types of leadership, sometimes with an argument that there is some historical progression to be seen in them and sometimes with a claim that these are techniques that any individual leader can adopt or drop when circumstances demand.

Underlying the taxonomies we can see two very different assumptions about leadership: 1) leadership is a matter of personal characteristics (traits) of the leader; and 2) leadership is about social processes. One attractively minimalist summary of the second type of understanding of leadership identifies four common themes in the way leadership has been conceived: 1) leadership is a process; 2) leadership involves influence; 3) leadership occurs in a group context; and 4) leadership involves goal attainment. Leadership, therefore, can be defined as 'a process whereby an individual influences a group of individuals to achieve a common goal' (Northouse, 2004: 3, cited in Bolden, 2004: 5).

So now the 'leadership styles': there are many lists to choose from, though there is plenty of overlap. We want to warn the reader that like almost any taxonomy, styles of leadership are in some sense a fiction. They exaggerate difference to the point of stereotype in order to add to the sense of order and sometimes there is an implicit preference for some styles over and against others.

Our first taxonomy comes from Simon Western's 2008 *Leadership: A Critical Text*. It offers a useful introductory overview. As the title of his book suggests, he is not promoting any particular style of leadership. In fact he uses the term 'leadership discourses' to emphasise that he is describing first and foremost how leadership has been talked about and conceived rather than how it is actually practised or able to be practised. His 'four discourses' are:

- the leader as a controller;
- the leader as a therapist;
- the leader as a messiah;
- the eco-leader.

He describes these discourses as emerging from particular periods of recent history though continuing to have some influence. For example, the first, he says, can be traced to the notions of 'scientific management' promoted by industrialist F.W. Taylor, after whose ideas 'Taylorism' was named, in the early twentieth century. This emphasises efforts to maximise efficiency and control in order to increase output. The project of scientific management is to be ever more efficient through measuring and controlling resources. Although this approach grew to be considered dehumanising, recent attempts to 'modernise' the public sector in the UK have seen a reversion to controller leadership, focusing on targets and 'command and control' to achieve greater outputs. 'Leader as therapist' can be associated with the human relations movement that emerged mainly during the 1960s. It works from the assumption that the fulfilled worker is also a productive worker. The therapist leader would focus on engaging workers in order to increase their motivation and personal commitment. This discourse is popular in the public sector and other people-focused organisations. Leadership development is dominated by the therapist discourse, often focusing on 'developing the self'. 'Leader as messiah', associated with ideas of 'transformational leadership' and culture control, arose from the 1980s onwards in the US. The aim was to create strong and dynamic cultures under the vision of a transformational leader. Loyalty and commitment within teams, and linking personal success to company success were key goals. Control is achieved via peer and self-surveillance, rather than hierarchical power or coercion. Finally, 'eco-leadership', the most recent phenomenon, emphasises connectivity and interdependence both within an organisation and beyond its boundaries.

For other categorisations let us return to so-called leadership 'traits'. First, we should remember that the concepts of character 'traits' has been developed by psychologists rather than sociologists. In this book we are using, broadly speaking, sociological theory to make sense of social phenomena. So we are trying to examine how, in this instance, psychological ideas have been used to support and promote certain social practices in organisations and specifically the health service.[2] In the 1970s the following list of character traits associated with leadership were identified (from a review of studies published at the time):

- strong drive for responsibility;
- focus on completing the task;
- vigour and persistence in pursuit of goals;
- venturesomeness and originality in problem-solving;
- drive to exercise initiative in social settings;
- self-confidence;
- sense of personal identity;
- willingness to accept consequences of decisions and actions;
- readiness to adsorb interpersonal stress;
- willingness to tolerate frustration and delay;
- ability to influence the behaviour of others;
- capacity to structure social systems to the purpose in hand. (Stogdill, 1974: 81)

It has to be emphasised, however, that the same set of traits has not been identified in other studies.

---

[2]Trait theory also underlies certain approaches to the currently fashionable 'values-based recruitment' discussed elsewhere in this book.

Here is another popular type of taxonomy of leadership styles:

Situational leadership: This developed from the late 1960s onwards and emphasises that an effective leader will be able to alter their style of leading in response to the situation at hand and the task needing to be completed. One example would be that the skill and maturity level of subordinates influences the way the leader leads. High skill and maturity level staff might call for a coaching and supporting approach from a leader while low skill and maturity is likely to call for more directive and delegatory approaches. Are you aware of this in the way that you have been treated by qualified staff or managers? Have you noticed this in the way that healthcare support workers are managed? See the later section in this chapter.

Transactional and transformation leadership: These are often described in contrast to one another, a clue that they may be idealised positions rather than descriptions of day-to-day work. Perhaps they can be seen as points on a continuum. Transactional leadership is said to be founded on the simple transaction between leader and subordinate of pay and security in return for effort and reliability. 'Transformational' leadership on the other hand emphasises the leader's ability to change the hearts and minds of followers in a way that identifies a moral dimension and challenge to the work at hand and empowers and excites followers to rise to that challenge.

Charismatic leadership: We have already outlined an early approach to this idea of leadership. It can be understood as a blend of the trait approach with the transformational model – the individual 'born to lead' and with the ability to motivate and change their followers. The idea of charismatic leadership, while still popular, has come under criticism. Some 'charismatic' business leaders have turned out to be at the heart of financial and other scandals while others rapidly move on from the organisation that they have exercised charisma within, leaving behind a range of problems needing to be solved. Some say this problem has afflicted parts of the NHS.

Distributed leadership: this model proposes that individuals at all levels in an organisation, not just those with formal management titles, and in all kinds of roles can exert leadership influence over their colleagues and thus influence the overall direction of an organisation. Distributed leadership is a more collective concept and refocused from the individual leader's qualities to an identification of what makes for effective and appropriate leadership processes within an organisation, a shift from attention on managers to everyone within the organisation (see Bolden, 2004).

Finally, you might be wondering whether the story of political and business leadership is largely a story of men. Many writers have pointed out the low representation of women in powerful and influential positions. For example, of the 500 largest US businesses less than 5 per cent have female chief executives. Likewise there are only 19 female elected leaders in the world (Llopis, 2014). Many have asked whether women lead in different ways to men and there is an often repeated assertion that women are better at people-centred, emotionally intelligent aspects of leadership, though there is little research to support this. Where there is research, it tends to concern perceptions about men and women in leadership and management. For example US researchers claim that studies suggest that:

the characteristics people typically associate with leadership are often stereotypically masculine. In particular ... *agentic* traits – conventionally masculine descriptors such as 'assertive,' 'forceful,' 'dominant,' and 'competitive.' These masculine traits are more likely to be viewed as characteristics of a successful leader than stereotypically feminine *communal* traits like 'affectionate,' 'compassionate,' 'warm,' and 'gentle.' ... The alignment of the stereotypical characteristics of men and the stereotypical characteristics of good leaders makes it easier for men to be perceived as successful leaders ... In contrast, women are perceived as less fit for leadership because traditionally feminine characteristics are less consistent with our perceptions of successful leaders. (Eagly and Koenig, 2014)

We will talk about women in leadership in the NHS a little later in this chapter.

Leaders and managers: what is the difference between the two?

Most texts about leadership ask this rather rhetorical question, rhetorical because the people who pose it often already have a position that makes the answer predictable. The distinction that most writers have made generally reflects the difference between Weber's bureaucrat and charismatic leader. The manager, according to these definitions, may be appointed to a position in an organisation and may develop 'leadership' skill whereas the leader is recognised by the people around them as providing leadership irrespective of their organisational office. Some have said that the manager 'does things right' while the leader 'does the right thing'. Others have said that management is about coping with complexity while leadership is about initiating and coping with change. The mere fact of having been put in charge (for example as a nurse being put 'in charge' of the ward for a shift), as many say, does not automatically confer leadership status. Your experience to date in the health service, we imagine, has already confirmed this. More recent writing about leadership and management is clearer that the contrast between the two, as well as the widespread implicit preference for 'leadership', does not reflect how people actually work in real jobs.

Most of us have become so enamoured of 'leadership' that 'management' has been pushed into the background. Nobody aspires to being a good manager anymore; everybody wants to be a great leader. But the separation of management from leadership is dangerous. Just as management without leadership encourages an uninspired style, which deadens activities, leadership without management encourages a disconnected style, which promotes hubris. And we all know the destructive power of hubris in organisations. (Gosling and Mintzberg, 2003, cited in Bolden, 2004: 7)

Reflection 8.1

Bring to mind any nurse you have come across who is a manager – either of a community team or in a hospital ward. As a thought experiment see if you can make separate lists of their 'management' and 'leadership' functions. A typical management function might be to be responsible for devising duty

> rotas while 'leadership' could be considered to be representing the interests of the ward/unit to those higher up in the organisation or setting an example of high standards of practice to those in the team.
>   Is either list longer? Is either list harder to make?

Our final point, which will bring us neatly to a focus on leadership and management in the UK's NHS and within the nursing profession, concerns power and coercion. It could be that power and coercion represent the blind spots of much organisational writing on this topic. As we have mentioned, most leadership texts draw on a list of generally unprovocative religious (Mother Theresa) and political figures to illustrate the attractiveness of strong leadership, but some highly effective and charismatic leaders never make it into these lists. This includes Adolf Hitler (Third Reich Germany), Joseph Stalin (Soviet Union), Saddam Hussein (Iraq) and the leaders of various religious cults. The justification for their exclusion is sometimes the argument that they are tyrants, rather than real leaders, whose goal is self-interest and not the interests of those they lead. In one sense this is right. Business leaders do not tend to have the ability to order the deaths of their rivals, though friendly Western political leaders certainly have. They can, however, taking the founder of Apple Inc. Steve Jobs as an example, initiate summary dismissals and public humiliations of employees and wield the power of highly changeable despots. In addition, as anyone who has come across a charismatic leader will know, the distinction between self-interest and concern for the advancement of an organisation or team is sometimes impossible to make. The business literature on leadership is often silent about this built-in ambiguity.

A second point concerns power. Much of the development of ideas about leadership originates from the model of the commercial world, where to a large extent – certainly larger than in the public sector – executives are able to wield more uncompromised power. Leadership and management in the UK NHS is very different, far more constrained and under constant internal challenge from professional groups and a level of outside 'interference' (as some would see it) from politicians that would be untenable in the world of business. So it is to this complex world, the world that you are now part of, that we turn.

Leadership in healthcare

Leadership in today's sense was first promoted in the UK NHS in the mid-1980s, during the period of Margaret Thatcher's government. Traditionally, right-wing governments in the UK have been more impatient with the welfare sector than their left-wing opponents because the welfare state is generally seen as a creation of the left. However, if you have studied modern-day UK politics you will be aware that this left–right dualism no longer applies in the same way that it did 60 years ago. The contemporary right critique of the NHS has been on two grounds. First, that it has exemplified a negative version of the features of bureaucracies described earlier.

With such an orientation to the office rather than the office holder and the separation of most individuals' work from personal reward, the service as a whole has become like a vast and slow machine with no one taking responsibility for guiding its overall direction or for initiating change and improvement. In the market vocabulary of the 1980s to the present day, the NHS has showed little responsiveness to its customers and operated for its own convenience rather than that of those who use or rely on the service. Just one example would be the practice of issuing the same appointment time to the entire list of an outpatient clinic and then the clinic start being delayed because the doctors that it relies on are scheduled to undertake previous work that regularly overruns. The ground of the second critique also concerns doctors, and to a lesser extent nurses and other clinical professional groups. If, when the NHS was set up in 1948, it could be considered a bureaucracy, it was a bureaucracy with a difference in that it was largely, if not formally, run by the medical profession. That profession, like all professions (see Chapter 3 'Becoming a nurse') offers an orientation and a loyalty that is separate from the particular organisations in which its members chose to work. The argument has been that doctors involved in the NHS had little incentive to be responsible for the judicious management of resources and were able to make a series of decisions – to initiate new expensive treatments for example – with little concern for their financial and other resource implications, for example the requirement for the employment and training of a new range of support staff associated with that treatment. The result was that the total cost of the NHS, as well as the configuration of services within it, grew in an unplanned and increasingly unaffordable way.

Enter, in 1979, the Conservative government of Margaret Thatcher. Her novel approach was to stop focusing on levels of absolute funding for the NHS and to start talking instead about *efficiency*. As the daughter of a grocer, it seemed appropriate that her government chose the head of the large supermarket chain Sainsbury to lead an inquiry into the management of the NHS. The 'Griffiths report' was released in 1983 and the NHS has never been quite the same since. Roy Griffiths in that report famously wrote: 'If Florence Nightingale were carrying her lamp through the NHS today she would be searching for the people in charge' (Griffiths, 1983: 12). Griffiths criticised a lack of accountability in the service and recommended the introduction of general management to replace the traditional tripartite system of separate management structures for doctors, nurses and administrators, the latter being widely seen as having the sole purpose of making the work of doctors run more smoothly. In response the government started recruitment campaigns to appoint strong and bright managers from the private sector and from the military. The clinical professions protested, as might be expected, on the grounds that no layperson could possibly manage (interfere with) the complex and highly skilled work of doctors and nurses. Hostility rumbled on and word has it that those few doctors and nurses who did successfully apply for management posts became despised by their clinical colleagues (Degeling et al., 2003).

In research I carried out in the early 1990s in NHS organisations in England, shortly after another reorganisation, I found that the bookshelves in chief executives' offices were full of the popular management paperbacks mentioned earlier. *In Search of Excellence* was particularly well represented. Some commentators saw the incorporation of professionals into management roles as an effective method of controlling professional activity:

In the 'old days' the NHS hospital could sometimes seem to exist for the doctors, rather than the other way round. Pre-Griffiths administrators saw their role as one of facilitating the work of doctors and nurses, not controlling or directing them. However, the contemporary ethos is much more one of the professional as a member of a team, and beyond that, of an employing organisation. The presumption is that the individual professional will be subject to the rules, plans and priorities of that organisation. (Harrison and Pollitt, 1994: 135)

The 1990s has been considered the era of the rise of managerialism, the introduction, or the attempt to introduce, management approaches and practices from the business world into the public sector – health, welfare and education among other areas. A 'managerialist' view would go something like this:

the world should be a place where objectives are clear, where staff are highly motivated to achieve them, where close attention is given to monetary costs, where bureaucracy and red tape are eliminated. If one asks how this is to be achieved the managerialist answer is, overwhelmingly, through the introduction of good management practices, which are assumed to be found at the highest pitch and most widely distributed in the private sector. (Pollitt, 1993: 7)

In the public sector during this time governments confronted the major professions and their key weapon was to put in place increasingly coercive management structures along with systems for measuring 'performance' along with 'naming and shaming' organisations or even individuals who appeared to depart too far from norms or fail to meet targets. However, the disadvantages of this approach have emerged recently with key reports into NHS problems tending to highlight the need for more collaborative forms of leadership where mistakes can be learnt from in a so-called no-blame culture (Berwick, 2013; West, 2014). A recent review of studies into management and leadership in the NHS shows that in practice 'hybrid managers', that is those individuals combining clinical and managerial roles, now outnumber general managers by four to one. But some long-standing problems still remain: while evidence shows that organisations that achieve high levels of engagement with clinical medical staff are more likely to perform well, levels of medical engagement vary considerably between healthcare organisations. Although there has been progress in involving doctors in management, continuing professional tribalism of managers, doctors and nurses and suspicion of those in hybrid clinical management roles still persists (NHS National Institute for Health Research, 2013).

Women and NHS leadership

As in many areas of public life and leadership, women are underrepresented in NHS senior leadership positions. The King's Fund (2013) noted:

While women make up three quarters of the NHS workforce, just 37 per cent of senior roles on clinical commissioning group governing bodies and NHS provider boards are held by women. Despite women making up 81 per cent of the non-medical workforce in the NHS, men constitute the majority in the leadership teams of all but just 12 per cent of providers and 10 per cent of clinical commissioning groups.

There are many programmes that have supported women to reach leadership positions in the NHS. At the time of writing, among them are the Athena programme (www.kingsfund.org.uk/leadership/leadership-development-senior-leaders/athena-executive-women) and the Mary Seacole programme (www.leadershipacademy.nhs.uk/programmes/mary-seacole-programme/).

Professional leadership in nursing

As we have seen, sociologists have studied the features and practices of professions largely separately from the study of bureaucracy, although they have some features in common; for example, both the bureaucrat and the professional are expected to make dispassionate decisions that put their clients' interests above their own and be impartial towards these clients. Given what we have discussed in this chapter, let's see how far we can separate organisational management from professional leadership.

Reflection 8.2

Ask yourself: 'So what might a nursing leader look like?' Here are some possible answers, features that might differentiate the nursing leader from the organisational manager – though of course many are (trying to be) both:

- Nursing leaders can, and do, articulate what nursing, and being a nurse, is about.
- They understand and share your professional aspirations and frustrations.
- Something about them – their behaviour and achievement – makes them role models.
- They argue the case for nursing resources and influence within organisations and in public.
- They are confident enough in their commitment to nursing to sometimes criticise it, if necessary, in public.

Can you think what else might characterise a nursing leader?

Many consider that good leadership at ward and clinic level is essential to maintain standards of patient care. It is probably not difficult to list, as above, desirable qualities and behaviours of these leaders. Nursing magazines are full of such lists and urgings to nurses to be better at them. However, professional leadership happens in a context and in certain contexts it becomes limited and even blocked. Before I give two examples from 'scandals' in NHS care, I want to make one point. Some readers might find this focus on failures makes depressing reading. However, my point is that if individual nurses are continually exhorted to perform better as a leader or as a nurse and the structural obstructions and difficulties they face are glossed over then it is likely that those individuals eventually blame any lack of impact on their own failure to try hard enough.

The 'Bristol Inquiry' was a wake-up call for medicine in the UK. The Bristol Royal Infirmary and the Bristol Royal Hospital for Sick Children were teaching hospitals that cared for patients, particularly small children with heart disease. Concerns were expressed about the mortality rate for some surgical procedures for babies with congenital heart disease. Complaints were made about certain surgeons to the General Medical Council and eventually two were struck off and another was disciplined. A public inquiry was opened in 1998. The report of the inquiry concluded that the cause of this failure was 'multifactoral and multidisciplinary' (Kennedy et al., 2001: 23); however, the report's authors have this to say about the nurses involved and about nurses in general:

> We regard it as significant that we did not hear concerns being brought to senior figures at the [United Bristol Healthcare NHS Trust] by the nursing staff. We do not infer from this any lack of concern on the part of nurses. Rather, we see it as illustrating a larger truth. The hierarchical system common at the time (and regrettably still too prevalent now) made it difficult for the nursing staff to voice concerns and to be heard. It is revealing that only when independent experts from outside the UBHT ... came to carry out their Review, did Fiona Thomas feel able to express her concerns about the lack of proper organisation in the ICU. It is also indicative of the state of affairs that the only way which Kay Armstrong and Mona Herborn felt was open to them to make known their dissatisfaction with aspects of [paediatric cardiac surgery] was to withdraw their services from the operating theatre when a Switch operation was to be performed. Nursing staff were let down by a culture that excluded them. (Kennedy et al., 2001: 175)

My second example of blocked professional leadership concerns the inquiry into peripartum hysterectomy at Our Lady of Lourdes Hospital, Drogheda, in the Republic of Ireland. This inquiry was called to investigate the reasons for an excessive rate of hysterectomies over a period of many years for young women, carried out by one obstetrician who worked there. The doctor in question was suspended and eventually struck off; however, one of the crucial questions that the inquiry asked was why this bad practice had been allowed to continue for so long. Some midwives had voiced concerns but no action had been taken. The judge who carried out the inquiry wrote:

> We tried to understand why the midwives, who formed the largest group of health professionals involved and who were principled women of training and intelligence, did not take their concerns further. Why did they not speak to management? Why did they not bring their concerns to the Matron and her assistant? ... The sad reality was that the Matron of the Maternity Unit was not given the power to properly administer the Maternity Unit. She lacked the authority necessary to question the consultants or to change procedures and she lacked the support of the [owners of the hospital] if a dispute arose ... Her long years working with the [hospital owners] moulded her into a caring and deeply committed, but submissive nurse with no confidence to take her concerns to a higher level, or to follow through on them. Many of the nurses we interviewed fitted the same mould. (Harding Clark S.C., 2006: 156–186)

What is the lesson for professional leadership from these extreme examples of probably more commonplace but less serious situations? To be effective, nurse leaders need not only to show the kind of characteristics and behaviours we listed above but to have equal organisational power alongside senior medical and general managers. The reasons that sometimes they do not have been discussed in this, and other, chapters. They involve long-standing differences in gender, class and professional power and influence. But society is changing and let us be optimistic that nurses and nurse leaders are increasingly able to practice their profession unblocked by these negative forces and with the support of initiatives that we mentioned earlier.

Delegation and the division of labour

> There are over 1.3 million frontline staff who are not registered nurses but who now deliver the bulk of hands-on care in hospitals, care homes and the homes of individuals. (Cavendish, 2013)

Increasingly the work of a nurse involves delegation of certain parts of the job to other workers. We want to end this chapter by talking about a sociology of delegation because delegation can be seen as a part of management and possibly leadership. As in many other areas of work, as nurses become more highly qualified and expensive to train and employ, the state and its managers give more attention to the division of labour. By 'division of labour' we mean something like this: 'the assignment of different parts of a task or manufacturing process to different people in order to improve efficiency' (*Concise Oxford English Dictionary*, twelfth edition, 2011: 419). It is well known that since perhaps the 1980s the 'tasks' of healthcare have been progressively passed from more expensive workers to those with less training (Allen, 2001). Nurses do the work that once was carried out by junior doctors such as giving intravenous drugs or prescribing medicines. Healthcare support workers do the work that recently was carried out by nurses such as bathing patients and recording vital signs while unpaid carers and patients themselves increasingly are given responsibility for tasks that used to be done by paid workers. So this constant shifting shows how the boundaries between professions are dynamic. We suggest that this changing division of labour and delegation can be looked at from three perspectives: economics, identity and trust.

Reflection 8.3

It takes five–six years to train a doctor and basic training costs approximately £274,000. Nurses take three years to train at an approximate total cost of something between £45,224 (Curtis, 2010) and £70,000 (Health Education England, 2013). The difference is partly due to the differential between the salary/bursary paid to medical students and student nurses, partly to the inclusion of tuition fees in the former cost and to the difference in cost of clinical placements. Assistant practitioners usually undertake a two-year foundation degree on a day a week basis. Healthcare support workers get hugely variable training, ranging from a matter of weeks to nine-month courses (Traynor, 2013: 64).

Looking at economics first, consider these two quotations (Allen, 2001). They are taken from the days of the introduction of Project 2000, mentioned elsewhere in this book, an approach to nurse education that was aimed to move from an apprenticeship model of training to a university-based approach, when student nurses became, for the first time, supernumerary. This change, like the more recent change to all-degree entry to nursing, pointed to a more highly qualified profession but it made governments start to realise that the nursing workforce could no longer be considered as a mass of inexpensive pairs of hands. That you might employ a smaller number of nurses to oversee and manage the work of a larger body of support workers becomes simply 'common sense' in the first quote from the then director of personnel for the NHS. His vision is a kind of industrial or managerial model of healthcare work as opposed to a professional one where the whole realm of the work would be controlled by members of the profession:

Project 2000 will bring out highly-trained professionals who we will have to use properly ... Nurses are locking themselves in too tight a definition. What's a doctor and what's a nurse? There's work to be done, you get the work done by the people who are best qualified to do it ... Hands-on care is below nurses' level of competence. The nurse will become the overall assessor of the care that the individual needs to have ... A higher quality cheaper service with a competitive edge will be achieved by those who make the most improvement in their labour costs. It's just common sense. (Eric Caines, Director of Personnel NHS, interviewed in 1990, quoted in Allen, 2001: 1)

The professional counter-argument, voiced shortly after the statement above, is this:

It may appear that many nursing activities can be performed by untrained people ... Nurses use bathing, washing and other forms of personal care) ... to perform other vital activities. Bathing is an ideal opportunity for observation of the skin and pressure areas. Counselling, reassurance and health education are carried out in a variety of settings when patients are relaxed and feel able to talk. Replacing trained nurses with untrained ones wherever possible will save money in the short term, but will prevent trained nurses having the vital and regular informal contact with patients and will affect the quality of total holistic care that nurses strive to deliver. (Rosemary Gillespie, letter to the *Guardian*, 15 May 1993)

The battle over skill-mix (what proportion of registered staff to support workers is needed and what number of registered staff are needed for any given number of patients) is still alive today and over the years it has taken many twists and turns. The days of high austerity and drastic cuts to the NHS staffing budget have been followed by the sobering warnings of the Francis Report (Francis, 2013) and the subsequent requirement (not widely implemented) for NHS wards to publish the number of qualified nurses on duty at each shift, with the profession itself arguing for a minimum ratio of patients to each registered nurse (Ford, 2013). Professions can take two approaches to this issue. First, they can push for increased numbers of members of their profession, as we have seen recently, and this argument has had some degree of success. For example in 2013, the BBC reported that Parliament's concerns regarding the quality of healthcare had shifted from a focus on training and values on to the numbers of nurses being employed in the NHS and nurse–patient ratios sufficient to ensure safe care (Triggle, 2013). Using workforce statistics from the Health and Social Care Information Centre, the BBC showed that in 2013 the number of nurses employed in England had fallen by about 3,000 (in full-time equivalents) since the Conservative/Liberal Democrat coalition came to power in 2010. The Royal College of Nursing has claimed that 20,000 unfilled nursing posts existed in England and that 'Unsafe staffing levels have been implicated in a number of high profile investigations into patient safety' (Dreaper, 2013). Shortly afterwards *How to Ensure the Right People, with the Right Skills, are in the Right Place at the Right Time* was published (Chief Nursing Officer for England and National Quality Board, 2014) giving guidance about levels of nurse staffing. More recent English NHS statistics show that the number of full-time equivalent nurses (excluding those employed by GPs) rose by 1.6 per cent between 2013 and 2015, and by 5 per cent since 2004. However, the number of support workers employed rose by 3.8 per cent from 2013 to 2015 and by 13 per cent since 2004 (Health and Social Care Information Centre, 2015).

In addition to campaigning for increased or, in a climate of reductions, maintained numbers of qualified staff, professions can emphasise their status by working to secure their control over some subordinate group, sometimes referred to as 'paraprofessionals' (Nancarrow and Borthwick, 2005). In the case of nursing, the paraprofessionals in question are healthcare support workers (sometimes known as healthcare assistants – HCAs) and their slightly more qualified colleagues assistant practitioners. We point to two pieces of evidence that this attempt has been made. The first is that the Royal College of Nursing has gradually drawn this growing group into full membership from 2001 onwards. In 2011 the RCN voted to enable HCA and assistant practitioner members to become 'full' RCN members and to take up seats on the RCN's governing council. (For further details see www.rcn.org.uk/hca.) The second piece of evidence is that training for these support workers is largely undertaken by nurses and, where these workers attend university for some of their training, by schools of nursing (Traynor et al., 2015). This involvement has sometimes been used as an opportunity to 'educate' support workers regarding their assisting role to nurses and to warn them not to think of transgressing the boundary between the two occupations (Allen, 2001).

The shifting boundaries between professions, however, can pose a threat for professional identity and, as we have seen, professional groups have a great deal invested in their distinctiveness for policy-makers and politicians, the general public and for members of the profession themselves. If there are financial and managerial pressures on nursing to delegate more of its traditional work with patients to support workers, there are contradictory (though perhaps fading) expectations from the public to maintain its image as the health profession with unique, close and caring contact with patients, and to act as 'patient advocate'. Nurses identify, formally at least, with the patient's interests. But with more direct patient care being undertaken by assistant/support workers and nurses increasingly taking on supervisory roles, the assistants themselves are starting to claim that they have taken over this privileged position while nurses, according to some of them of them we interviewed, become 'pen-pushers' (Traynor et al., 2015). So division of labour and delegation is ambiguous for nursing – it can both enhance a profession's standing to have a layer of subordinate workers to delegate potentially low-status work to[3] but it can threaten the identity of the profession if it is seen as giving away its core work to another group. To try to prevent this, the profession delegating work might emphasise the routine nature of that work and their overall supervisory position – 'having nurses give intravenous drugs, under the protocol we have devised, allows us doctors to concentrate on the real work of diagnosis and treatment of difficult cases'. In order to maximise the identity benefits and minimise the dangers the profession receiving such tasks might emphasise the opportunity to add an extra procedure to its repertoire – 'being able to prescribe a range of drugs allows us to provide more holistic seamless care and avoids patients having to wait for doctors to be available'.

Now, finally, let's consider trust and with it get to the heart of delegation. Both the nursing profession's professional body and the regulator have acknowledged that delegation to support workers is firmly on the map and both have been providing guidance on the topic for nearly ten years. The same challenges face many other healthcare professions and the guidance from the RCN was jointly issued with the Royal College of Speech and Language Therapists, the British Dietetic Association and the Chartered Society of Physiotherapy (RCSLT et al., 2006). This guidance takes the opportunity to emphasise that most integral of professional qualities, professional judgement: 'Choosing tasks or roles to be undertaken by support staff is actually a complex professional activity; it depends on the registered practitioner's professional opinion' (p. 4). The Code of Conduct produced by the Nursing & Midwifery Council (NMC, 2015) also includes a section on effective delegation and this consists of three requirements:

> only delegate tasks and duties that are within the other person's scope of competence, making sure that they fully understand your instructions; make sure that everyone you delegate tasks to is adequately supervised and supported so they can provide safe and compassionate care, and; confirm that the outcome of any task you have delegated to someone else meets the required standard. (p. 10)

The key problem is one of trust. And it is a problem because healthcare support workers or assistant practitioners are an unknown quantity. The proliferation of titles they go under and the lack of standardised training, not to mention the often-repeated fact that they are unregulated, differentiates them, on paper at least, from

---

[3]Some have explained the development of nursing in mid-nineteenth-century Britain as at least partly in response to medicine's need for 'a new type of support worker' (Gabe and Monaghan, 2013: 161).

qualified nurses. It means that delegation will almost inevitably proceed cautiously and on an individual basis. The overall competence of the support worker, broken down into individual competencies relating to specific abilities, should in theory form the basis of delegation. However, research has suggested that the character of delegation, and hence of the roles of these workers, depends, perhaps not surprisingly, on the subjective response of the nurses who manage them. One study described the approach to delegation between qualified nurses and support workers as use, misuse and non-use: misuse described situations where the support workers were used in ways that were 'beyond the expectations of formal policies and was described ... as "exploitation of the ... role" ...'. Non-use was exemplified by RNs 'preventing HCAs from putting their skills and experience into practice', for example not involving them in discussions about patient care (NHS Education for Scotland, 2010: 27). The same review goes on to summarise: 'Evidence suggests that the introduction of HCAs has been met with scepticism by a number of qualified staff who regard them as a cheaper alternative which have encroached on their role and territory' (ibid.).

The policy attention given to support workers has heightened since the publication of the Francis Report as well as the exposure of other healthcare scandals that have involved both support workers and nurses. It led the UK government to commission the subsequent Cavendish Review in 2013. With the government already rejecting the call for national regulation of support workers, the review recommended a nationally designed but locally implemented Certificate of Fundamental Care, now known as the Care Certificate. The bodies that were given responsibility to develop this focused explicitly on the issue of trust:

> The Care Certificate **IS** [original emphasis] the shared health and social care training and education which must be completed and assessed, before new HCSW/ASCWs can practise without direct/line of sight supervision in any setting. (Skills for Health, Health Education England et al., 2014)

This astonishing quote shows just how difficult it is to organise a service without trusting those engaged within it and it also shows, in our view, the frankly unrealistic expectation placed on nurses, and support workers themselves, to never be out of each other's sight until the support worker has successfully completed the 15 parts of the Care Certificate. Lack of trust in organisations can lead to complex arrangements of monitoring and supervision that according to some can cause a paralysis of inaction (Bachmann, 2001). It is no wonder that, according to many practising nurses and support workers, the latter's management and delegation is largely based on an informal and individualised trust.

Chapter summary

This chapter has taken as its starting point the emphasis on leadership – in both its good and bad forms – in recent writing about the NHS. Management has been the key mechanism that governments have used to achieve their aims for the service but it has also come in for sustained criticism in reports into NHS failings.

Leadership and management in society at large as well as in organisations has been studied by sociologists for over 100 years and has been the basis more recently of a huge industry promoting particular individuals' ideas and perhaps exaggerating the importance of management practices. Such ideas have been influential at various points in the NHS history, contributing to the rise of 'managerialism'. We have considered concepts such as bureaucracy and charisma as well as some of the very many typologies of management and leadership 'styles'.

The NHS is a complex arena for management and leadership for two reasons: first, because the service is highly politicised and targets, inspections and constant reorganisation are used by governments in attempts to try to solve its problems and shortcomings; second because its staff is highly professionalised and professionals tend to look to their own values and leaders for motivation and identity, seeing 'general' managers as over-concerned with financial requirements and lacking humanity.

Women may make up around 90 per cent of the nursing workforce, but they are underrepresented in senior NHS leadership positions. Nurses in corporate positions sometimes struggle to represent what they would consider nursing values in board-level decisions.

As nurse managers manage nurses, so staff nurses, including the newly qualified, are expected to 'manage' support workers by delegating suitable work to them and checking that it is done properly. Whether we like it or not, nurses are increasingly going to be supervisors of core 'nursing' work. So, in that sense, we are all managers now. And it is important to understand some of the critical sociological background to leadership and management today.

Going further

For a definition of and further details about critical management studies see www.critical management.org/ for links to critical management resources.

References

Allen, D. (2001) *The Changing Shape of Nursing Practice: The Role of Nurses in the Hospital Division of Labour*. London: Routledge.

Bachmann, R. (2001) Trust, power and control in transorganizational relations. *Organization Studies* 22(2): 337–365.

Berwick, D. (2013) *A Promise to Learn – A Commitment to Act: Improving the Safety of Patients in England (Berwick Review into Patient Safety)*. London: National Advisory Group on the Safety of Patients in England.

Bolden, R.I. (2004) *What is Leadership?* Leadership South West Research Report 1. Exeter: University of Exeter, Centre for Leadership Studies.

Cavendish, C. (2013) *The Cavendish Review: An Independent Review into Healthcare Assistants and Support Workers in the NHS and Social Care Settings*. Available at: www.gov.uk/government/uploads/system/uploads/attachment_data/file/236212/Cavendish_Review.pdf (accessed 6 October 2015).

Chief Nursing Officer for England and National Quality Board (2014) *How to Ensure the Right People, with the Right Skills, are in the Right Place at the Right Time: A Guide to Nursing, Midwifery and Care Staffing Capacity and Capability.* London: NHS England.

Curtis, L. (2010) *Unit Costs of Health and Social Care 2010.* Canterbury: Personal Social Services Research Unit.

Degeling, P., Maxwell, S., Kennedy, J. and Coyle, B. (2003) Medicine, management, and modernisation: a 'danse macabre'? *BMJ* 326(7390): 649–652.

Dreaper, J. (2013) Union claims nursing hit by 'hidden workforce crisis'. BBC News 12 November. Available at: www.bbc.co.uk/news/health-24874326 (accessed 6 October 2015).

Eagly, A. and Koenig, A. (2014) Research reveals how stereotypes about leadership hold women back. *Women at Work.* Available at: http://footnote1.com/research-reveals-how-stereotypes-about-leadership-hold-women-back/2015.

Ford, S. (2013) Nurse campaign calls for minimum 4:1 staffing ratio. *Nursing Times*, 11 June. Available at: www.nursingtimes.net/nursing-practice/specialisms/management/nurse-campaign-calls-for-minimum-41-staffing-ratio/5059580.article (accessed 20 May 2015).

Francis, R. (2013) *Report of the Mid Staffordshire NHS Foundation Trust Public Inquiry: Executive Summary.* London: House of Commons. HC 947.

Gabe, J. and Monaghan, L. (eds) (2013) *Key Concepts in Medical Sociology.* London: Sage.

Gerth, H. and Wright Mills, C. (eds) (1997) *From Max Weber: Essays in Sociology.* London: Routledge.

Griffiths, R. (1983) *Report of the NHS Management Inquiry.* London: Department of Health and Social Security.

Harding Clark S.C., M. (2006) *The Lourdes Hospital Inquiry: An Inquiry into Peripartum Hysterectomy at Our Lady of Lourdes Hospital, Drogheda.* Dublin: TSO.

Harrison, S. and Pollitt, C. (1994) *Controlling Health Professionals: The Future of Work and Organisation in the NHS.* Buckingham: Open University Press.

Health and Social Care Information Centre (2015) *NHS Workforce: Summary of Staff in the NHS: Results from September 2014 Census: Medical and Dental, Non-Medical and GP Censuses.* London: Health and Social Care Information Centre.

Health Education England (2013) *New Education and Training Measures to Improve Patient Care.* Leeds: NHS [updated 28 May 2013; cited 13 August 2015]. Available at: www.hee.nhs.uk/hee-your-area/north-west/news-events/news/new-education-training-measures-improve-patient-care.

Kennedy, I., Bristol Royal Infirmary Inquiry and Great Britain Dept. of Health (2001) Learning from Bristol: The Report of the Public Inquiry into Children's Heart Surgery at the Bristol Royal Infirmary 1984–1995. Norwich: The Stationery Office.

Keogh, B. (2013) *Review into the Quality of Care and Treatment Provided by 14 Hospital Trusts in England: Overview Report.* London: NHS.

King's Fund (2013) Women continue to face barriers to taking senior leadership positions in the NHS, new research finds. Press release. Available at: www.kingsfund.org.uk/press/press-releases/women-continue-face-barriers-taking-senior-leadership-positions-nhs-new 2015.

Llopis, G. (2014) The most undervalued leadership traits of women. *Forbes Leadership.* Available at: www.forbes.com/sites/glennllopis/2014/02/03/the-most-undervalued-leadership-traits-of-women/2015.

Nancarrow, S.A. and Borthwick, A.M. (2005) Dynamic professional boundaries in the healthcare workforce. *Sociology of Health and Illness*, 27(7): 897–919

NHS Education for Scotland (2010) *The Development of the Clinical Healthcare Support Worker Role: A Review of the Evidence.* Edinburgh: NES.

NHS National Institute for Health Research (2013) *New Evidence on Management and Leadership.* Southampton: Health Services and Delivery Research Programme.

NMC (2015) *The Code: Professional Standards of Practice and Behaviour for Nurses and Midwives.* London: Nursing and Midwifery Council.

Peters, T. and R. Waterman (1982) *In Search of Excellence: Lessons from America's Best-Run Companies*. New York: Harper and Row.

Pollitt, C. (1993) *Managerialism and the Public Services*. Oxford: Blackwell.

RCSLT, BDA, RCN, CSP and Trent RDSU University of Sheffield (2006) *Supervision, Accountability and Delegation of Activities to Support Workers: A Guide for Registered Practitioners and Support Workers*. CSP, RCSLT, BDA, RCN. Available at: http://www.rcslt.org/docs/free-pub/Supervision_accountability_and_delegation_of_activities_to_support_workers (accessed 6 October 2015).

Skills for Health, Health Education England and Skills for Care (2014) *The Care Certificate: Assessor Document*. Health Education England, Skills for Care and Skills for Health.

Stogdill, R.M. (1974) *Handbook of Leadership: A Survey of Theory and Research*. New York: Free Press.

Traynor, M. (2013) *Nursing in Context: Policy, Politics, Profession*. Basingstoke: Palgrave.

Traynor, M., Nissen, N. Lincoln, C. and Buus, N. (2015) Occupational closure in nursing work reconsidered: UK health care support workers and assistant practitioners: a focus group study. *Social Science & Medicine*, 136–7: 81–8.

Triggle, N. (2013) Nurses: the engine of the NHS. BBC, 18 September: www.bbc.co.uk/news/health-24142611 (accessed 1 April 2014).

West, M. (2014) Michael West: collective leadership – fundamental to creating the cultures we need in the NHS. http://blogs.bmj.com/bmj/2014/05/28/michael-west-collective-leadership-fundamental-to-creating-the-cultures-we-need-in-the-nhs/2015.

Western, S. (2008) *Leadership: A Critical Text*. London: Sage.

9

Using a sociological framework to understand nursing

Helen Allan,
Daniel Kelly, Pam Smith,
Michael Traynor

Introduction

This chapter doesn't start with a single issue. Instead we draw together some thoughts on the relevance of sociological theories to current nursing practice. In this book we have argued that nursing is fundamentally a social process involving interactions between people (patients, nurses, other members of the healthcare team) which takes place within socially constructed contexts that are determined by factors often outside the control of patients and nurses themselves. These social contexts shape the way that students are educated and enter the profession as well as how they undertake nursing work within the social structures of the nursing profession and National Health Service (NHS) organisations. They also, in turn, shape to a large extent how nurses deliver care in response to patient need. We have presented a range of analyses of contemporary nursing and healthcare issues which may assist you to better understand the complex social and interactional processes that make up your work as a nurse

We have argued that although nursing is unavoidably social it is often under-stood as predominantly biomedical. Of course it is essential for nurses to have a sophisticated understanding of the physiological, pharmaceutical and biomedical aspects of nursing care. However, in our view, these disciplinary approaches to health and illness offer an incomplete and insufficient basis upon which to provide nursing and to work effectively for patients in an organisation. Patients are clearly more than the sum of biological processes; moreover, the nursing and healthcare staff who deliver care to them work within a set of interconnected social conditions and structures that determine how that care is organised and delivered. These conditions and structures need to be understood before the physiological, pharmaceutical and biomedical aspects of patient care required to be undertaken to improve patient outcomes can be effectively delivered by nurses as healthcare team members. We have stressed the importance of understanding the dynamics that exist between social structures and individual agency throughout the book.

Our intention in writing this book is to look to the discipline of sociology to propose a framework, or set of frameworks and theories, to help you understand the complexities of modern nursing and healthcare. We have arrived at our understanding of the potential importance of sociology to the practice of nursing care through our own experiences of nursing practice, education and research. We have drawn on some of these experiences to provide practical examples of how sociology is relevant to nursing in the 'issues' which begin each chapter.

Chapter outline

Our intention in this chapter is to provide some concluding thoughts on each chapter and then reflect on some cross-cutting themes identified across the chapters. We also give you some strategies to deepen your understanding of the relevance of sociology to nursing and nursing practice.

Themes from each chapter

In the Introduction, we introduced you to the idea that you as an individual are shaped by the society, the social structures, the social networks and arrangements in which you live. These social arrangements and the social interactions or processes you engage in are the focus of the discipline of sociology. We emphasised that being aware of these social constraints or forces was relevant for understanding and nursing the patient with more insight. We introduced two important concepts: macro and micro approaches to sociological theory.

Chapter 1 dealt with how healthy people learn to become patients; we explained that sociological theories have shown how, once ill, patients are expected to behave in specific ways. We considered in some detail the doctor–patient relationship and the *sick role* as an example of macro-sociological theory; then we considered some critiques of this approach and a short analysis of power in the patient–nurse relationship;

before introducing micro approaches to the doctor–patient relationship such as symbolic interactionism, labelling and narratives or patients stories.

In Chapter 2 we considered illness as a social issue, and who were more likely to become patients; in other words, what particular social circumstances made it more likely that some people were more likely to become ill than others. We introduced the concept of health inequalities and considered some macro- and micro-sociological explanations for these health inequalities across social classes and over time.

Chapter 3 discussed how student nurses become nurses through a consideration of socialisation theories and in particular professional socialisation. This chapter also discussed what is meant by the term profession and why membership of these occupational groups is so highly prized. The chapter also gave an introduction to the concept of professional regulation.

In Chapter 4 we focused on sociological analyses of care work or caring by nurses and discussed their importance in relation to nursing as *women's work*, which is then underpaid and undervalued against equivalent men's work. We also considered some of the strategies nurses use to resist, assert and overcome domination, oppression and scapegoating.

Chapter 5 developed these ideas of caring to consider the emotional aspects of care work through the theories of emotional labour and face-work. In this chapter we introduced you further to the sociological concepts of structure and agency to consider how the nurse learns to manage his/her emotions and to prevent emotional burnout.

In Chapter 6 we considered that the reality of care work means caring for someone else's bodily and emotional needs. We considered different ways of conceptualising the body in nursing over time and introduced you to different approaches to understanding the effects of this work on nurses themselves.

Chapter 7 considered what happens when nurses are unable (or unwilling) to deliver safe or satisfactory standards of care and what some of the sociological explanations are for poor nursing. Although these concerns are highly topical in 2015, the recent reports into poor nursing care outlined in this chapter are not isolated incidents; care work is inherently difficult and constrained by both structural factors, such as workplace cultures, as well as individual agency.

In Chapter 8 we considered leadership and management discourses in nursing and healthcare more widely; we considered the conflicting interests nurse managers might be subject to.

Cross-cutting themes in thinking sociologically in nursing

We have identified four cross-cutting themes which we now address:

1. Working with others: context and behaviour
2. Thinking critically
3. Understanding nursing and healthcare management
4. Confidence to respond to scandals involving nursing.

Working with others: context and behaviour

Sociological frameworks are, at the risk of tautology, fundamentally social because they deal with the understanding of society-based phenomena. They offer explanations of human action that avoid the purely individual and individualistic. Our intention in writing this book has been to provide a sociological framework as the basis to working with patients and their families. Such a framework emphasises how people and groups find meaning in experiences such as illness or death and how this can often be very different to the meanings that healthcare professionals have developed about the work they do. Knowledge of this essential difference between the professional and the lay perspective can help you to explore what meanings patients and their families might make about health and illness. It can also enable you to understand the responses and behaviour of the patients you meet and so help you to deliver more effective care. Bringing a sociological view to nursing we have suggested might help avoid 'blaming' or stigmatising a patient. It is easier sometimes to 'blame' the patient for not adhering to a treatment regime, say not to give up smoking, instead of thinking through what might have been the social conditions that led him or her not to accept or be able to follow health advice. It is our view that understanding the complexities in healthcare, in patients' everyday lives, can help you understand patients rather than become defensive, cynical or 'burnt out'.

As well as working more effectively with patients we suggest the material that we have presented in this book will give you an understanding of how healthcare systems operate, from the level of the hospital ward or community clinic to the function of a whole organisation and the nation's healthcare service as a whole. Praise for success and blame for failure in nursing and healthcare tend to be directed at individuals or certain groups (in the case of failure to care, this has been nurses who don't care anymore), but a sociological understanding can show us, for example, how 'failure' was almost inevitable in the way that a system – or ward – has been set up as a result of various forces operating upon it at a political or societal level. In short, a sociological understanding may lead you to avoid 'blaming the victim' and, crucially, blaming yourself for system-wide failures (as we discussed in Chapter 7).

Sociology also provides an understanding, or set of understandings, of the historical and contemporary forces acting on health professions; including their differential status and the character of their interactions, which are often shaped by social or gender-based differences in power. Even an elementary understanding of these factors can enable you to develop a more informed, sophisticated and effective approach to working with different nursing colleagues as well as members of other professions who make up the healthcare workforce (as discussed in Chapters 3, 4 and 8).

Thinking critically

Another intention in writing this book is to encourage a habit of thought that questions taken-for-granted assumptions – whether they are involved in professional work or education for a single professional role – and to examine these assumptions critically, in this case through the lens of sociological theory. It is our experience that being critical in nursing is sometimes difficult or resisted, especially when work is busy and the workforce is put under pressure to keep within targets, get through the work or to solve particular problems (as discussed in Chapter 7). The critical thinker will ask 'For whom is this really a problem and for what reasons?' or 'Why is this happening here and now?'

We hope the material we have presented has also helped you to be equally critical and analytical of the experience of being a student in today's UK university system. As we have seen, much writing about socialisation in nursing contrasts the university setting with the workplace, identifying the former with the transmission of positive values. The critical thinker will ask, 'In what way is the system of nurse education and the forces that shape the curriculum unhelpful for developing the confident, questioning practitioners that the profession claims to want?' (as discussed in Chapter 3).

Understanding nursing and healthcare management

In this book we have provided what we have found to be helpful insights into leadership and management in nursing and healthcare. We hope we have provided you with a range of theories that will help you understand the rewards and incentives that managers have to work with, for example, as these may not be always communicated clearly in the busy and sometimes hierarchical context of the NHS. We also hope we have given you a sophisticated understanding of the *talk* often used when referring to nursing leadership in the NHS (see Chapter 8). This understanding will help in your work as a staff nurse and later if you choose to become a manager, to manage resources and your team effectively and humanely.

Confidence to respond to scandals involving nursing

Our intention in writing this book has also been to assist students to respond to the scandals involving nursing. We have been asked frequently by our students, what do you think of the Francis Report? This book is one of our responses as a group of experienced nursing academics who have enjoyed diverse careers in nursing. Throughout the book, we hope to have shown that understanding the crises and various issues that are challenging the profession – and the NHS more generally – *sociologically* helps to reveal how complex these issues and challenges actually are and how much they need to be thought about carefully. Looking for simple solutions or blaming one group of workers alone (a response often favoured by politicians of the day) may seem attractive but will ultimately prove inherently futile as responses to complex problems need to draw on a mix of research evidence, theory and experience and utilise each wisely. We hope that this ability to reflect thoughtfully by drawing on sociological theories will help you enter into debates with your colleagues – or even publically – in an informed and more confident way (see the reference to the grumbling appendix blog in Chapter 3).

Some nurses are reluctant to engage in such debates and find them discouraging; however, we highlight throughout this book that healthcare problems do not go away simply by ignoring them. It is our view that such problems require a thorough analysis before solutions can be imagined and developed to address them. This is true from national 'problems' to local and team-based problems with individual patients or families.

Conclusion: strategies to help you think sociologically and become a more reflective, critically minded nurse

In writing this book, we have argued for the necessity for the future nurse to be critical, analytical, and informed by sociology as well as physiology, psychology and pharmacology, confident to respond to critiques of current nursing and able to work effectively whilst being aware of how the social context of work effects patients, their families, themselves and other healthcare workers equally.

This book is intended as an introduction to sociological theories, the thinkers behind them, sociological debates, key sociological concepts and ways of thinking. We hope reading it will have whetted your appetite to study more sociology and think further about how it applies to healthcare, illness and nursing as work. You might go on, as we did, to develop research careers or, as practising nurses or as nurse leaders, continue to be research-minded so that you can be critically minded in practice and provide, as far as you can, care that has some basis in research evidence. As you know from your own academic work as a student, research mindedness often involves learning about or deepening your understanding of sociological and other concepts. This can be part of acquiring understanding of research methods – from survey research to phenomenology – or of developing sociological understandings and theories with which to interpret research data. This understanding, in turn, can help you, and those who read and assess your academic work, to understand how to deliver more effective care to patients as well as provide helpful insights into the delivery and organisation of that care with an acute awareness of the power of workplace cultures.

Nursing work is complex, exciting, satisfying and sometimes overwhelming. We hope our book offers you the intellectual tools to rise to the challenge of understanding this complexity and to make the most of what can be a uniquely challenging but fascinating 'sociological' career.

Index